Theory in Health Promotion Research and Practice

Thinking Outside the Box

Patricia Goodson, PhD
Professor
Department of Health & Kinesiology
Texas A&M University
College Station, Texas

JONES AND BARTLETT PUBLISHERS
Sudbury, Massachusetts
BOSTON   TORONTO   LONDON   SINGAPORE

World Headquarters

Jones and Bartlett Publishers	Jones and Bartlett Publishers	Jones and Bartlett Publishers
40 Tall Pine Drive	Canada	International
Sudbury, MA 01776	6339 Ormindale Way	Barb House, Barb Mews
978-443-5000	Mississauga, Ontario L5V 1J2	London W6 7PA
info@jbpub.com	Canada	United Kingdom
www.jbpub.com		

Jones and Bartlett's books and products are available through most bookstores and online booksellers. To contact Jones and Bartlett Publishers directly, call 800-832-0034, fax 978-443-8000, or visit our website, www.jbpub.com.

This publication is designed to provide accurate and authoritative information in regard to the Subject Matter covered. It is sold with the understanding that the publisher is not engaged in rendering legal, accounting, or other professional service. If legal advice or other expert assistance is required, the service of a competent professional person should be sought.

Production Credits

Publisher: Michael Brown
Editorial Assistant: Catie Heverling
Editorial Assistant: Teresa Reilly
Senior Production Editor: Tracey Chapman
Associate Production Editor: Kate Stein
Senior Marketing Manager: Sophie Fleck
Manufacturing and Inventory Control Supervisor: Amy Bacus
Composition: diacriTech
Art: diacriTech
Cover Design: Kristin E. Parker
Printing and Binding: Malloy, Inc.
Cover Printing: John Pow Company

Library of Congress Cataloging-in-Publication Data

Goodson, Patricia, Ph. D.
    Theory in health promotion research and practice : thinking outside the box / Patricia Goodson.
        p. ; cm.
Includes bibliographical references and index.
    ISBN-13: 978-0-7637-5793-9 (pbk.)
    ISBN-10: 0-7637-5793-4 (pbk.)
    1. Health promotion—Philosophy. 2. Health promotion—Research. I. Title.
    [DNLM: 1. Health Promotion. 2. Health Planning. 3. Models, Theoretical.
WA 590 G655t 2009]
    RA427.8.G66 2009
    613—dc22
                                                                        2009015393
6048

Printed in the United States of America
13 12 11   10 9 8 7 6 5 4 3 2

Dedication

This is dedicated to my father, Rev. Curtis C. Goodson, and his wife, Elisa G. Goodson, with much love.

Contents

Preface

It never fails. Every time I begin teaching a health behavior theories course—before students have had a chance to learn what theoretical thinking entails—I hear the familiar mantra: *"But, Dr. Goodson, theory is sooooo boring, sooooo dry, and sooooo abstract!"* (with lots of emphasis on the "so" to make sure I don't miss the point). Despite their preconceptions that learning health behavior theories is as enticing and exciting as hiking through the Saharan desert in the middle of a sand storm, they concede, rather reluctantly at first, that theory may be a needed (often required) tool for health promotion. If so, then learning how to use it *might*, indeed, be valuable. Yet mastering this tool seems as unattractive a task as undergoing brain surgery (or any surgery, for that matter).

It is for readers who identify with such prejudices against theory, who believe theory is dry, boring, and unappealing, that I wrote this book. Because I do understand why people might think this way about theory (yes, I concede: theory *can be* a horribly abstract and unattractive topic), I wrote *Theory in Health Promotion Research and Practice: Thinking Outside the Box* as a different kind of theory book. Because I wanted readers to actually enjoy reading about theory, this book *had to be* different.

What, then, makes this text unique? First, it does not describe any particular theory or sets of theories used in health promotion research or practice. I wished to avoid the book becoming a mini-encyclopedia of theories, for plenty of such resources are readily available. I even present and assess some of these resources within the text (see Chapter 4).

If it does not describe individual theories then, what is the book *about?* The answer to this question is rather simple: The book centers on a *challenge*—a challenge I propose to you, the reader and health promotion professional (or professional-in-training), to develop your theoretical thinking skills in order to impact the field, improve people's health, and foster professional growth. Across all chapters you will find a constant, repeated call to think theoretically, to develop your own theoretical frameworks, to fill in the current theoretical gaps, and to enjoy yourself in the process! This is, most certainly, the main purpose of this book—its "soul."

More specifically, *Thinking Outside the Box* is about the need for and the importance of *thinking theoretically* about health promotion and public health. Chapters 1 and 2 define theory and develop a rationale for why thinking theoretically is vitally important for the health of our field (very frequently, I will use the labels "health promotion," "public health," and even "health education" interchangeably, despite their inherent differences). Chapter 3 reviews how health promoters (scholars and practitioners) have handled theoretical thinking and the application of theory to research and practice in recent years (or not). Chapter 4 introduces you to the available textbooks describing the various health education and health behavior theories currently employed in the field (the mini-encyclopedias I mentioned previously). The chapter exposes you to the theoretical landscape that our health promotion efforts now inhabit, and offers to take you through a *theoretical-thinking journey*, critically assessing the most popular theories we employ in public health research and practice. The journey takes you through Chapters 5, 6, and 7, pointing to three important problematic patterns in the current landscape: current theories' exaggerated focus on individual-level factors, their undue emphasis on rationality, and their deliberate privileging of linearity.

Before you begin to fear *Thinking Outside the Box* might just be a heavy-handed critique of the theories currently deployed in health promotion, I remind you of the book's main title: *Theory in Health Promotion Research and Practice.* That is precisely the topic I address in Chapters 8 and 9, providing guidelines for *applying* theory (yes, those same theories I critique in Chapters 4 through 7) to health promotion research (Chapter 8) and to program planning and evaluation (Chapter 9). Keep in mind: In Chapter 8, you will find step-by-step guidelines for applying theory to the three most-often employed research paradigms in public health— quantitative, qualitative, and mixed-methods research. If, for some reason, you picked up this book merely to learn how to *use* theory, you may want to read Chapter 1 (for the overall "tone" of the book) and skip to Chapters 8 and 9 (and Appendices A and B) to get to the procedural steps.

In Chapter 10, you will find "outside-the-box" recommendations for bridging the gap between theory and practice in public health. Appendix A provides a brief overview of the distinction between *theory* and *model*, and in Appendix B, I offer brief guidelines for how to develop your own theoretical thinking, and how to evaluate the quality of a new (or even an "old") scientific theory.

Thinking Outside the Box is a different kind of theory book not only due to its content. It is different because it proposes a unique way of thinking *about theory*. In this text, I argue that thinking theoretically is essential for reflection about one's practice and is, therefore, a *type of practice* itself. I also make the case for theoretical thinking as *narrative*, for theories as *stories*, and for theorizing as a form of *story telling*. These notions—that theory is practice, that theory is a form of narrative—are not new. Yet they represent an uncommon approach to theoretical thinking, one that sits at the margins of the current scientific discourse in public health, one you will not encounter very frequently in public health's arsenal. While these perspectives may currently lack widespread popularity, I believe them to be the most interesting (not boring), attractive (not dry), and effective (not irrelevant) approaches for helping to understand the professional dilemmas we face and the many frustrations we encounter when dealing with human beings, their well-being, and dis-*ease*. I encourage you not to be deterred by the nonmainstream status of some of the perspectives I introduce; after all, that's what thinking outside the box entails—becoming part of a minority group of thinkers.

To support the unconventional approach I bring to this book (yet I must remind you that the approach is unconventional mainly in public health, not so much in other fields), I relied heavily on the authors who have shaped my own theoretical thinking. I attempted to reflect their views through my own lenses of personal and professional experiences. Among those who influenced my approach to theory and theoretical thinking, the Brazilian educator and philosopher of education, Paulo Freire holds a prominent place (partly because I had the privilege of hearing him speak several times at conferences in Brazil and was fortunate to have been mentored by a couple of his closest pupils—one of whom became Freire's biographer). For those unfamiliar with Freire's work, it may suffice to know that he is viewed as the "father" of empowerment theories in health promotion.

I agree with Freire's basic premise that education is a powerful transformational tool. If I didn't believe this, I wouldn't have chosen *health education* as a career. Yet it is his specific formulation that education is a *dialogical process of action and reflection* that became the foundation of my thinking about health promotion research and practice. For Freire, all education occurs within a process of dialogue between free human beings. In this dialogue, humans exchange and create meaning (or *teach-and-learn*) by "naming" the world around them. The words used in this naming process come from the work (or praxis) that humans engage in, work they do to transform and manage their world. This work consists necessarily of two dimensions: reflection and action. These dimensions interact so radically, claims Freire (1974), that "if one is sacrificed—even in part—the other immediately suffers" (p. 75). When, in human praxis, action is sacrificed, what results is *idle chatter, verbalism* or, as Freire would say, an "*alienating 'blah.'*" Conversely, if reflection is compromised, human action turns into *nervous activism* and shuts down dialogue. In other words, too much action—without reflection—is nonceasing activity without room for meaningful dialogue; too much reflection—without corresponding action—becomes empty babbling and has no transformative power (Freire, 1974). According to Freire, in our educational and knowledge-building efforts, we are constantly tempted to break up this reflection–action unit and to dichotomize (and polarize) the two dimensions. Such dichotomy—established in most disciplinary fields, including public health—between theory and practice, action and reflection, is concrete evidence that we have fallen into temptation. But more about that later in the book.

A third reason why this is a different kind of theory book is its writing style. Precisely because I believe education consists of an ongoing dialogue between teachers and learners, I opted to write this book using a "dialogue tone": I write the text, as much as possible, in the first person, something you will not find in most theory texts. Because I wished to maintain a conversational style and avoid some of the "dryness" of other theory texts, I tell several stories of my interactions with colleagues and students, their puzzled questions, their reactions, and their experiences applying theory (or not). I confess I received mixed reviews when a few students read the initial drafts of this book. Some asked that I avoid the "I" in the text; for them, using first person became too distracting and did not make the text sound "academic enough." "Stick to the facts and write academically" was their somber advice to me at that point, perhaps feeling an obligation to protect my career from abject disaster were I to continue insisting on writing informally. On the other extreme were the students who "absolutely *loooooved*" the personal, informal style and thanked me profusely for avoiding writing another text that might significantly increase the risk for a reading-induced coma. Go figure. Mixed reviews! As an academic, shouldn't I be used to them by now?

Backed by Robert Nash—and his text *Liberating Scholarly Writing: The Power of Personal Narrative*—I chose to err on the side of mixing "much informal writing with formal writing" (Nash, 2004, p. 6). Actually, I *had* to, you see, because this book defines, discusses, and assesses theory from the perspective of narrative, or theory-as-story telling. This approach compels me to write in a style that allows interspersing my own stories, inserting my own voice. Granted, I don't have *that many* interesting stories to tell related to theory; so I did break down and "stuck to the facts" at least 90% of the time. Yet you will catch me breaking the rules of academic discourse quite frequently in each of the chapters. I hope you won't charge me with academic mutiny and will instead become motivated to explore what Robert Nash calls "scholarly personal narrative"(SPN). Nash defines SPN as a form of intellectual inquiry that advocates, for the inquirer, the author, or the researcher, the right to be placed *inside* the exploration, to have his or her voice heard *alongside* the "mere facts" (Nash, 2004, p. 4). I strongly believe in the intrinsic value of this type of inquiry.

This text was written for graduate students and junior professionals who work directly with or have a tangential interest in human health and well-being, public health, and health promotion; students in schools of Public Health; in departments of Health Education, Human Behavior and Performance, or Health Promotion; within colleges of Education or Health Sciences; and those enrolled in human health behavior-related studies in Anthropology, Sociology, Psychology, Political Science, and Social Work (among other fields). I believe the text will also be useful for public health professionals who might feel twinges of frustration every now and then regarding the prosaic theoretical direction in which the field seems to be headed, who wish to contribute new perspectives and approaches, who wish to think "outside the box" yet not feel completely alone or unvalidated in the process. Ultimately, this book can represent a source of solace and direction for anyone wishing to navigate the theoretical waters in the social sciences.

If you find the text helpful (or even if you don't) and wish to share your comments, provide feedback, ask questions, or recommend changes, you're welcome to email me at ***TheoryDoc@gmail.com***. I look forward to hearing from you.

REFERENCES

Freire, P. (1974). *Pedagogy of the Oppressed* (M. B. Ramos, Trans. 10th printing ed.). New York: The Seabury Press: A Continuum Book.

Nash, R. J. (2004). *Liberating Scholarly Writing: The Power of Personal Narrative.* New York: Teachers College Press.

Acknowledgments

During the journey I undertook writing this text, I learned it takes a village to place a new book in readers' hands. I am fortunate to inhabit a village teeming with talented, tenacious, and tactful supporters, readers, reviewers, editors, and publisher. My gratitude extends to all fellow villagers, but I would like to single out a few people who deserve special recognition. First and foremost, the editorial, production, and marketing teams at Jones & Bartlett Publishers, where 90% of the people assigned to work with me were named "Katie" (what are the odds?). Thank you, Katey Birtcher, who held my hand at the beginning of the contract-signing and writing processes; Catie Heverling, Editorial Assistant, who walked me through the production–launching steps with much grace and patience; Kate Stein, the production editor; and Sophie Fleck, the marketing manager, for kindly answering all of my basic (often very naïve) questions. I actually had fun through this process that most authors find "grueling" and "boring." I learned a lot from each of you. My most sincere thank you to Michael Brown, Publisher, for believing in the value of this project and providing a review of the final product that was absolutely on target! Thanks, Mike!

I am also grateful to Texas A&M University for granting me a Faculty Development Leave in the spring semester of 2008; it represented concerted writing time away from the numerous interruptions inherent in teaching, mentoring, directing research projects, and exercising administrative tasks. Texas A&M University also represents a big portion of my village, and I wish to extend a sincere thank you to the colleagues there who encouraged and supported this project. Among them are Dr. Buzz Pruitt, who knew this book just "had" to be written, no matter what; Dr. Carolyn Clark, who held my hand during the Faculty Development Leave and often reminded me, "You will finish the book!"; Dr. Yvonna Lincoln, who fostered the necessary confidence to approach a publisher with the idea for this book in the first place; and the students in various health behavior theories classes in my department who read the first chapters of the book and provided valuable feedback. A special note of thanks goes to my faithful P.O.W.E.R. group at Texas A&M.[1] I never expected the group would provide such valuable support for my own scholarly writing! That group is the best!

Several colleagues and friends at other universities (my extended villages) also deserve special recognition. A world of thanks to Dr. Debby McCormick, at Northern Arizona University, for cheering this project along, for just loving Chapter 5 in its draft format, and for keeping me humble during the process (she has a knack for doing that!). A big thank you is also in order to my former students, now assistant professors in their own right, who read selected portions, commented, or eagerly volunteered to adopt this text: Dr. Eric R. Buhi, Dr. Lei-Shih Chen, Dr. Heather Honore, Dr. Sandra Suther, Dr. Adam Barry, and Dr. Catherine Rasberry.

I also received invaluable support in the form of emotional strength and encouragement from two nonacademics (but true educators, at heart). One of them is my chiropractor and acupuncturist, Dr. Karen Campion. I do not manipulate the truth (no pun intended!) by saying this book would never have been written were it not for her patience and dedication in taking care of my "out-of-whack Qi." ("Qi" is a Chinese term meaning body–soul energy.) Her gentle, healing hands are a testament to alternative therapies and to the effectiveness of an energy–medicine approach to health promotion. The second nonacademic is my electrical engineer turned-missionary father (now retired), to whom I dedicate this text. His unwavering belief that this book was worth writing and his steadfast commitment to listening to my reports of progress, set-backs, and accomplishments were invaluable; they represented a tangible sign of true grace and made me so very thankful.

These are the villagers who helped make this book a reality. They are worthy of thanks and recognition, but are not responsible for any mistakes or idiosyncrasies I may have brought to the text. Together, we would like to invite you to be a part of this village and to come stay awhile and commune with us as you read. . . . We are thankful you chose to visit. We hope you enjoy your stay.

Patricia Goodson
College Station, Texas
TheoryDoc@gmail.com

---

[1] I created P.O.W.E.R. services, in 2007, as a peer-led service to support doctoral students' writing efforts in the College of Education and Human Development at Texas A&M University. P.O.W.E.R. stands for Promoting Outstanding Writing for Excellence in Research.

About the Author

Patricia (Pat) Goodson, PhD, is a Professor in the Department of Health & Kinesiology at Texas A&M University, where she has taught many of the graduate-level health behavior theories courses during the last 10 years. She obtained her PhD in Health Education from The University of Texas at Austin (thankfully, Texas Aggies do not hold that against her!). She holds one master's degree in General Theological Studies, awarded by Covenant Theological Seminary (in St. Louis, Missouri), and another one in Philosophy of Education, from the Universidade Catolica de Campinas (in Campinas, São Paulo, Brazil). Dr. Goodson's bachelor's degree in Linguistics, her bilingual (Portuguese-English) and bicultural upbringing, and her interest in all things language-related have converged in the narrative approach to theory and to health promotion that she brings to this book. In addition to this text, Dr. Goodson has authored several publications related to her research interests in reproductive health, human sexuality, sexuality education, and public health genomics. You may contact Dr. Goodson at: *TheoryDoc@gmail.com*.

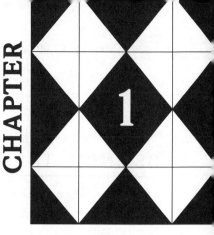

CHAPTER 1

Theory as Practice: Thinking Theoretically About Health Promotion

Learning Objectives

When you finish reading this chapter, you will be able to:

1. Describe similarities between commonsense and scientific theories.
2. Choose a definition of scientific theory that makes the most sense to you.
3. Articulate a definition of theoretical thinking (or theorizing) and theory.
4. Further examine and test the notion of theories as stories.
5. Outline what theory/theorizing does.
6. Articulate the concept of theory as practice.
7. Question why the unity of theory-practice is often broken in public health.

. . . There is nothing so practical as a good theory.
—*Kurt Lewin, 1951*

DEFINING THEORY

I *love* theory because, really, there's nothing more practical! Yet it took me a long while to truly appreciate the practical side of theorizing because when I began studying health behavior theories I felt I had been trapped within a dream-like, bizarre world in which everything seemed disproportionately abstract. I had a hard time understanding precisely what a theory *was*, what exactly it could do to guide my research, and how on earth I would even *know* which theory to use. My difficulties began when attempting to define theory, as I could never uncover a simple explanation: scholars' conceptualizations and explanations were so abstract, convoluted, and complex that I often gave up trying to craft a definition of my own (and did I mention how *confusing* it all seemed?).

Eventually, I came to think of "what is theory?" as an unimaginative question: on one hand, presupposing simplistic, reduced accounts of a seemingly rich phenomenon and, on the other, offering abstract, complicated, and unintelligible answers. After all, one's impulse is to fill in the blank in "Theory is (blank)" with a quick, concise, one-sentence description, but the concise and short definitions I came across rendered theory meaningless, lifeless, confusing, and (to quote my students) "awfully dry."

A friend of mine enjoys reminding me that "theory is not rocket science; it's much more complicated than rocket science!" If this holds true, then it doesn't sit well to define theory as one single, simple entity. As I came to understand much later in my studies, theory is multifaceted and amazingly complex. To reduce it to a one-dimensional phenomenon would come close to mutilation, and as you see throughout this text, theory's beauty lies precisely in its dynamic and intricate complexity (Hoffman, 2003). Brief definitions never do it justice.

If asking "what is theory?" leads nowhere interesting, I believe it more productive to ask a different set of interconnected questions such as these:

- What does theory do?
- What does theory—in action—look like?
- How can we recognize theory when we see it?
- What does theory do that is uniquely "theory-*ish*"?

Although this book, as a whole, addresses all these topics, I have chosen to center this chapter on the first two questions, relating them specifically to the world of health promotion and public health:

1. What does theory do?
2. When theory is doing its "thing," what does it look like?

The most common approach to health promotion theories found in your professional materials (books, journal articles, reports, websites) goes as far as admitting that theories have at least two faces or may be found in two different varieties (but rarely more than two): *commonsense theories* and *scientific theories*. As you read along, you will find this book introduces you to other types of theory, but for now, let's begin by considering these familiar categories and then proceed with answering the two questions I proposed previously.

Commonsense Theories

Commonsense theories comprise explanations we invoke, on a daily basis, to make sense of our lives. For example, in the past couple of weeks, Laura's behavior seems a little "off." She arrives late for team meetings and appears distant and broody when the team interacts. Laura is one of my graduate assistants and doctoral students. I do have a "theory" (or a proposed explanation) for Laura's behavior: She has been under considerable stress lately, taking her comprehensive exams, finalizing a manuscript to submit for publication, and teaching two freshmen-level classes.

My theory is a "commonsense" theory because it represents a personal attempt to make meaning of a situation (a sense-making task), based on the information at hand. I may choose to test this theory of mine, for instance, by asking Laura herself if what I'm thinking is valid or by asking some of her colleagues about what is happening, but such testing won't go far: As soon as I understand what is going on or as soon as her behavior returns to "normal," I will forget my little theory and the need to test it and will gladly move on to the next problem.

Another good example of commonsense theories is conspiracy theory. You can certainly recognize a conspiracy theory when you see one: It tends to grab your imagination. Conspiracy theories combine challenging questions with sometimes outlandish answers, attempting to explain why something happened. Take President John F. Kennedy's assassination, for instance. Many explanations have been proposed to make sense of the bizarre events that ended the President's life.

Among these explanations, a handful of conspiracy theories have emerged. These theories started by zeroing in on the questions that were dismissed or brushed aside by the mainstream official reports because they (the questions) were unthinkable, outrageous, or too far fetched (the theory proposing that President Kennedy and Governor Connally were not struck by a single bullet is only one example of the many conspiracy theories that sprung up after the event) (Kurtz, 2006).

Frequently, unique perspectives or approaches are followed, and unusual solutions to difficult problems are sometimes found, thanks to these conspiracy-type accounts, but yes, you're quite right if you thought about this: Very often, conspiracy theories find themselves unsupported by available evidence and, with time, become tales and myths societies enjoy telling and retelling.

Yet, underlying both commonsense and conspiracy theories you find a shared element: attempts to make sense of reality, to explain events and circumstances so humans can function in a world, in a reality, in a place furnished with meaning.

Scientific Theories

Scientific theories, as you have already noticed throughout your studies, look different from commonsense theories from the get-go. Definitions of scientific theories are much more elaborate, contain more clearly outlined characteristics, and have better defined purposes when compared with definitions of commonsense theories. Here are some examples of these definitions as they appear, specifically, in the social sciences. In the now-classic textbook on health behavior theories, *Health Behavior and Health Education*, for instance, theory is defined as "a set of interrelated concepts, definitions, and propositions that present a *systematic* view of events or situations by specifying relations among variables, in order to *explain and predict* the events or situations" (Glanz, Rimer, & Viswanath, 2008, p. 26).

Another elaborate, yet a bit clearer definition of social science theory is proposed by Norman Denzin (1970):

> A theory is a set of propositions that furnish an explanation by means of a deductive system. *Theory is explanation.* Durkheim's theory of suicide in Spain conforms to the above specifications. . . . It states that: (1) In any social grouping, the suicide rate varies directly with the degree of individualism (egoism); (2) the degree of individualism varies with the incidence of Protestantism; (3) therefore, the suicide rate varies with the incidence of Protestantism; (4) the incidence of Protestantism in Spain is low; (5) therefore, the suicide rate in Spain is low. (p. 34, emphasis mine)

Here are other definitions providing further details regarding scientific theory's main elements:

> A theory is a set of interrelated universal statements, some of which are definitions and some of which are relationships assumed to be true, together with a syntax, a set of rules for manipulating the statements to arrive at new statements. (Cohen, 1980, p. 171)
>
> Theory is a mental activity. . . . It is a process of developing ideas that can allow us to explain how and why events occur. Theory is constructed with several basic elements or building blocks: (1) concepts, (2) variables, (3) statements, and (4) formats. (Turner, 1986, pp. 4–5)

In our world of public health, health education, and health promotion, "behavioral theories are composed of interrelated propositions, based on stated assumptions that tie selected constructs together and create a parsimonious system for explaining and predicting human behavior" (DiClemente, Crosby, & Kegler, 2002, p. 3).

When examined further, these definitions also refer to scientific theories' three main goals, purposes, or functions:

1. *Description.* Theories should facilitate the description (and understanding) of the phenomena being studied. The scientist/social scientist must be able to "describe the phenomena he [sic] is studying so that others can repeat his descriptions with a high degree of agreement" (Denzin, 1970, p. 31).
2. *Explanation.* Scientific theories allow "the construction of a system of interrelated propositions that permits the scientist to 'make sense' out of the events observed" (Denzin, 1970, p. 31).
3. *Prediction.* The utility of scientific theories extends beyond mere description and explanation, however. "If a [scientist/social scientist] claims to have explained why a given set of variables occurs together, he must be able to predict the future relationships" (Denzin, 1970, p. 31).

This, in a nutshell, is how scientific theories are often defined and characterized.

As you examine these accounts, what would you say is the common theme cutting across all of these definitions? What is similar about them? Yes, the notion that scientific theories explain phenomena in a logical, ordered, interconnected manner. As we found for commonsense ones, scientific theories also represent attempts to make sense of reality, through descriptions, explanations, and predictions of events and circumstances.

From the previous set, my favorite definition is the one proposed by Turner (1986, p. 4), for it places theory in the world of words or ideas (a mental activity), highlighting the power of language to create and shape human reality (if ever you had any doubts about the power language has in creating and shaping reality, just read J. R. Tolkien's *Lord of the Rings*, J. K. Rowling's *Harry Potter* series, or Robert Frost's poems).

Not far from my top choice for a good definition of scientific theory is Cohen's (1980, p. 171) proposition, because his includes an important characteristic of scientific theories. To earn the status of "scientific," theoretical explanations need to go together, connect according to specific rules, and follow a unique grammar. Denzin (1970) calls this set of rules, or this grammar, a "deductive system." Explanations of cause and effect, by themselves, do not constitute a theory. They are merely explanations. What lends these explanations the status of theory is the manner in which the explanations are connected, derived from, or related to each other. Here, Denzin (1970, p. 34) puts the same idea differently: "A theory must contain a set of propositions or hypotheses that combine descriptive and relational concepts. . . . Unfortunately, a set of propositions taken alone does not constitute a theory either. The set must be placed in a deductive scheme."

This particular feature of scientific theories (relationships among explanations or constructs) reminds me of quilting. If you've ever tried your hand at this craft, you know quilting consists of sewing fabric together, usually combining large squares of material with different textures and colors to form an intricate pattern. Quilting offers a very useful image for the process of theory building because you can "see" how, depending on the way you choose to connect the blocks of fabric, you can get entirely different images. For instance, take a look at the squares I drew in Figure 1–1.

The various designs displayed in the last row of Figure 1–1 were all formed by combining the top square into blocks of four squares each (shown in the second row). The variation in shape has everything to do with how the original block is combined with other identical blocks. The same goes for scientific theories: string the data (or "facts") using a certain logic or set of beliefs as the starting point, and you come up with one set of explanations; combine them within another (logic) structure (some like to label these structures *paradigms*), and the resulting explanations might look very different. The important point to remember from this illustration, however, is this: Individual blocks of fabric do not a quilt make. Similarly, you don't have a scientific theory until you weave various explanations within a logic pattern.

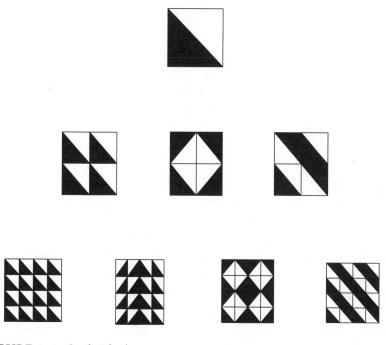

FIGURE 1–1 Quilt Blocks

So, there you have it: my two favorite definitions of scientific theories. Yet, if you do not agree with my choice and have your own preferred version(s), don't worry! You're in good company. Surprisingly enough, neither in the "hard" sciences nor in the social sciences do scholars share a single agreed-upon view of what a theory is, nor do they care to reach consensus over a single definition (Cohen, 1980; Turner, 1986). Although for some the term "theory" may refer to a "set of tested empirical generalizations" or to a "unified, systematic causal explanation of a diverse range of social phenomena" (Schwandt, 2001, p. 252), others may view theory as broad "theoretical orientations or perspectives (e.g., functionalism, symbolic interactionism, behaviorism)" or, more specifically, as a single theory (e.g., critical theory) (Schwandt, 2001, p. 252). At the same time, various types of ideas, speculations, hypotheses, models, criticisms, conceptual frameworks, or any propositions interconnected with words (and even scholars' personal beliefs) are sometimes called theory in certain disciplinary fields (Cohen, 1980; Denzin, 1970). Go figure!

Therefore, despite the apparent rigor, order, logic, and systematic thinking going on in scientific theorizing, social scientists themselves use the term theory to mean many different things. Far from indicating these scientists don't have their act together, to me, this only reinforces the notion that theory is a complex, multidimensional phenomenon that resists attempts to be simplified, unidimensionalized, and "boxed" into one specific container. The beauty of theory lies precisely in its intricate complexity, much like the beauty of a kaleidoscope, a fractal image, or the inner workings of the human body.

THEORIZING, THEORETICAL THINKING, AND THEORY

The way many health promotion (and social sciences) textbooks define and emphasize scientific theories is, to me, part of a plot (do you sense a "conspiracy theory" in the making, here?): A plot to simplify theoretical thinking, to reduce it to its bare bones, to "skeletonize" the phenomenon, and thus to distance us from the forces involved in its creation, implementation, and refinement. Perhaps it is merely an attempt to be didactic, not a plot. In trying to help us understand, textbook authors have instead taken us into an anatomy lab, made us look at a cadaver, and declared, "Here is what life looks like!" It just doesn't work for me.

The problem, as I see it, is this: Definitions of scientific theories ignore a crucial element within the theory domain—the theorizing *process*. To think about theory is to think about explanations, descriptions, and predictions, yes, but it is more than that. It means also considering the questions and the reasoning that lead to these explanations, descriptions, and predictions.

For my purpose in this book then, I define theorizing (or theoretical thinking) as the dynamic process of *asking and answering* specific types of questions. I define theory as the end result, the outcome, the outgrowth from this operation. Put another way, theorizing implies movement, dynamics, dialogue: a volleying between questions and replies. Theory is the answer part of the equation. You can see this conception of theory and theoretical thinking diagrammed in Figure 1–2.

Within this framework, scientific theories are characterized by questions focused on causes, with explanations or answers that attempt to tell the story of why phenomena occur as they do. Theoretical questions in scientific-type thinking about health promotion ask: What influences or determines healthy behaviors among older adults? Do attitudes lead to behavior change among adolescents? Why is education level associated with certain health outcomes? Scientific theories—when they have already been proposed and tested—provide clean, decluttered explanations to answer these questions. They have been carefully

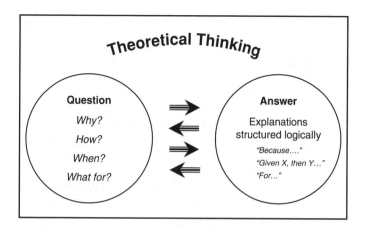

FIGURE 1–2 The Theorizing Process

thought out, tentatively proposed (at first), and repeatedly tested to see whether the explanations might hold over time and across various contexts. Only after much tweaking, adjusting, and testing, testing, testing do these explanations gain the status of a scientific theory, and, in science, all of the tweaking, adjusting, and testing follow carefully spelled-out protocols. In other words, they are done in a systematic way, following principles and procedures of scientific practice (Pedhazur & Schmelkin, 1991).

Other types of theories (policy, ethics, common sense theories) ask different types of questions. They are not cause-and-effect ones, but questions such as: What is the ultimate end of health promotion? Why should healthier lifestyles be promoted? Are the means being used to promote health, healthy themselves? Is health a human right to which all human beings are naturally entitled? How can a country's public health system protect its populations against potentially dangerous illnesses? What can be expected from the impact of globalization, in terms of health promotion, worldwide?

THEORY *AS* PRACTICE

What Does Theory Do?

Setting aside the differences between commonsense and scientific theories, I hope it has become clear to you that both categories have a pivotal, common element: meaning attribution. This is precisely the "job" of theoretical thinking. This is exactly what theory, or more precisely theorizing, does (Nealon & Giroux, 2003).

Theory-type questions and their answers lend meaning, provide explanation, impose order, and organize logically the events that engulf us. Theorizing, in other words, leads us to:

- *Ask* certain types of questions
- *Question* the status quo
- *Seek* the most plausible and meaningful answers
- *Build* a narrative or logical structure for the questions and the answers

We should view theory as a type of practice precisely because theorizing involves all of these actions. Just keep this point in mind: *theory is practice*. If practice is "action" or "doing," we find that theory does quite a lot more than we might suspect. So, the next time someone attempts to criticize you because you enjoy thinking theoretically, you can point out how thinking theoretically is, indeed, engaging in very practical tasks!

What Does Theory Look Like?

Remember the textbooks that—at most—propose two different "faces" for theory: commonsense and scientific? In order that you may grasp the unique characteristics of scientific theories, these books' authors will often draw a sharp distinction between the two types, almost to the point of suggesting they are incompatible or contradictory. The truth is if you view theoretical thinking as a process of asking specific types of questions and obtaining certain kinds of answers, scientific theories and commonsense theories become merely different manifestations, different "looks" of the theorizing process. Both appear different, but the difference is on the surface, in the types of questions raised. The bottom-line processes of sense making, meaning attribution, explanation, and description, remain the same for both types (for all types) of theories.

Many scholars defend the notion that humankind's most universal strategy for making sense of reality is that of creating and telling stories. "We are storied selves," says Robert J. Nash (2004, p. 8). Because theories are one way to explain and attribute meaning to reality, theories undeniably constitute a specific type of story (Hoffmann, 2003). Mark Edberg (2007) describes the notion well:

> It could be said that a key characteristic of modern humans from prehistoric times has been the creation of tales, myths, and stories that, for example, describe an entire cosmological system, explain the creation of society, explain how men and women came to be what they are, and so on. These are all theories in the broad sense, for they present a coherent account from which more specific judgments and conclusions can be drawn. (p. 26)

I would like to make this point clear. When Edberg or I say that theories are stories, we are not saying that theories are the product of fantasizing about make-believe worlds. We mean this: Theories themselves are built following certain narrative structures, certain "story-building rules" and purposes. What these stories or theories "look like" depends on whether they are scientific theories, public policy theories, ethics theories, commonsense theories, or conspiracy theories. Packaged in different formats, they all represent ways to provide accounts of phenomena in orderly, logical, and meaningful ways (Lemert, 1993). In this sense, theories are stories. Notice how Arthur W. Frank, author of *The Wounded Storyteller*, describes the book in which he analyzes the human experience of disease by focusing on his and others' personal stories of illness:

> This book [*The Wounded Storyteller*] is a *work of theory*, but it is equally a collection of stories and a kind of memoir. For almost a decade I have been a wounded storyteller, and I have cultivated the stories of others who are wounded, each in different ways. The "theory" in this book elaborates my story and theirs (Frank, 1995).
>
> Charles Lemert introduces his social theory textbook calling theory "a basic survival skill" (Lemert, 1993). *The Wounded Storyteller* is a survival kit, put together out of my need to make sense of my own survival, as I watch others seeking to make sense of theirs. The wounded storyteller, like Lemert's theorist, is trying to survive and help others survive in a world that does not immediately make sense. (p. xiii)

If stories are crafted and told for sense-making purposes (for survival, Frank and Lemert would say), however, they only have meaning within a given context. The Biblical story of the creation of the cosmos makes no sense within the context of physics and astronomy. Theories of health promotion that emphasize individual responsibility for wellness have little relevance in refugee camps, among victims of natural disasters, or among populations afflicted by wars. To understand what theory looks like or what kind of meaning it is creating, a theory must be understood within its particular context, against the backdrop of the particular stage in which it is enacted. Edberg (2007) puts it clearly:

> [Theories] are propositions that have meaning, validity, and truth (or falsity) within a specific context, such as a historical context, a social context, or a cultural context. Within their contexts, they are commonly held to be meaningful. Thus, to understand why a particular theory is meaningful or to evaluate its validity, you need to understand the contextual ground rules, so to speak. (p. 26)

Keep this point in mind: theories will "look" different, depending on the context within which you search for them. They will have unique appearances, depending on the needs they were designed to meet at the time they were created. Furthermore, they will only be considered "true," "valid," or even "useful" depending on the historical, social, and cultural circumstances within which they were invented.

If that context is the natural sciences in the 20th and 21st centuries, for example, theories will look very rigid, very authoritative, and some will have gained the status of "universal laws" (e.g., the law of gravity). In this context, the need being met is that of discovering realities existing outside human experience, of developing factual, predictable knowledge: hard-fast, lasting, and stable rules, efficient at prediction and control. On the other hand, if the context is the behavioral sciences within modern Western societies, theories will be numerous, varied, much more malleable, and almost none will have achieved the status of "universal" explanations despite much testing. Some of these theories will even question the theorizing or sense-making processes themselves, asking whether the search for meaning is, indeed, a universal trait among humans.

Within the context of behavioral sciences—lying at the intersection of biological and social sciences—the need being met by scientific theories is both to explain or "gain clarity" (Buchanan, 2004) regarding humans as individuals and social beings and to predict and control human behavior. If the context is public policy, theories will be less concerned with the ability to understand human behavior and more with facilitating healthy community living and protecting individuals within specific population groups. If the context is Western ethics, you will find theories focusing more on normative aspects of human lives (what should be done, what is ethically right or wrong) and providing guidelines for seeking out the common good.

The outcome of the theorizing process, therefore, as well as the theorizing process itself, will assume many "personas," for theories wear the clothing provided by their historical and practical contexts. Much in the same way that Tofu takes on the taste of the sauce in which you cook it, theories take on the form, shape, language, norms, and values of the many contexts in which they are built and applied.

Health educators tend to think of health promotion theories, quite often, as universally applicable scientific explanations about health behaviors. Public health in general and health education in particular could benefit substantially from investigating, in more depth, the contexts from which these health promotion theories have emerged and in which they are embedded. At the very least, understanding of these theories' historical and cultural contexts would allow health promoters to have realistic expectations about their (the theories') potential and limitations for 21st century public health practice.

THEORY *VERSUS* PRACTICE

In the fall of 2006, at the start of my "Behavioral Foundations of Health Education" class (an introductory, graduate-level health behavior theories course), I asked the students to jot down brief answers to this question: "What comes to mind when you hear the word 'theory'?" I told them I was looking for emotions, beliefs, descriptions, or definitions that immediately surfaced when they thought about the term.

Not surprisingly, of the 14 responses I collected, none listed a single positive emotion. Half contained what I considered neutral or descriptive elements (such as "relationship, explanation, ideas, hypotheses, logical process, concepts, road map"). The remaining half of the class, all of them, brought up negative or critical elements. Here are a few examples:

> Not factual
>
> Old—dating back many years and may or may not be improved or changed
>
> Hard to prove and understand
>
> Something abstract, difficult to understand
>
> Not useful
>
> Lack of concrete parameters and confusing guidelines/boundaries

Here is my favorite: "Theory is complex, something I don't like thinking about. . . . It's a lot of thoughts with no specific answers."

You don't need recounts of my students' beliefs (before they took my class, mind you!), however, to illustrate the negativity some people exhibit regarding theory. You find these same attitudes sometimes displayed in textbooks themselves. Here is an example of a preface to a well-known book on theory-driven evaluations (Chen, 1990):

> I would be more sympathetic to [the author's] use of "theory" if that term did not carry with it such a load of unwanted meanings. For example, in sociology, "theory" is often equated with the abstract essays written by sociologists who are long dead. In other fields, theory is equated with sets of integrated mathematical statements concerning highly abstract properties. (p. 9)

Several reasons lie behind the negative reputation theory currently enjoys, particularly in public health, and some are quite complex. I won't develop them in detail here, but in Chapter 3, you will come across a few explanations for why there is such a theory-practice misalignment in public health (and, as it turns out, in most other applied professions). An important possibility to consider, however, is this: Could it be that, specifically in public health and health promotion, the separation between theory and practice is so pronounced because scholars and practitioners have applied the *wrong types of theories* to the task of facilitating healthy decision making and behaving? In other words, is it possible that researchers or academics (the theorists) have been asking theoretical questions that are "not productive" for understanding why human beings do what they do? Could they perhaps be theorizing about human health behaviors by asking the "wrong" type of question? Theorists and researchers have insisted on asking what causes human behavior (in the same way they would ask what causes a certain cell to replicate or what causes a planet to maintain its orbit). Should they be asking questions about the purpose and the meaning of human behavior, instead (Buchanan, 2000)?

To help us ponder whether this might, indeed, be possible, I invoke Aristotle (and thank David Buchanan [2000] for making Aristotle's thinking so easy to understand). Theorizing (or philosophizing) about human knowledge, Aristotle classified human experience into three types, each type generating a specific kind of knowledge. Here is a small chart (Table 1–1) listing these experiences and resulting knowledge, which I drew based on the outline provided by Buchanan (2000, p. 54).

To this day, Western thinking about what knowledge is has been influenced by Aristotle's typology, and in a way, it is helpful to understand the multiple ways in which humans experience reality and learn from such experience. For Aristotle, episteme-type knowledge—or the type of knowledge we gain from observing "events that are constant, universal, and eternal" (Buchanan, 2000, p. 54), the type of knowledge being generated in the natural sciences—is

Table 1–1 Aristotle's Classification of Types of Knowledge Resulting from the Three Types of Human Experience

Types of Human Experience	Varieties of Knowledge Generated by Each Experience
Theoria: ". . . the experience of events that are constant, universal, and eternal."	Episteme
Poesis: ". . . the experience of making things—know-how or craftsmanship."	Techne
Praxis: ". . . experience [that] comes from the encounter with flux: the transient, irregular, context-bound, and contingent relationships characteristic of the sociohistorical domain."	Phronesis (or Practical Reason)

Data are from Buchanan, D. R. (2000). *An Ethic for Health Promotion: Rethinking the Sources of Human Well-Being.* New York: Oxford University Press. By permission of Oxford University Press, Inc.

"inadequate and inappropriate for analyzing social situations." As Buchanan (2000) explains,

> Aristotle observed that human relationships are historical, contextual, and contingent. Action in the social domain must be responsive to the novel features of each situation, to contexts in which a limitless variety of features fluctuate in salience, and to the ethical relevance of the particular persons in the specific situation at hand. (p. 54)
>
> While the force of gravity is uniform throughout the known universe (except, possibly, in black holes), Aristotle noted that relationships in the sociohistorical domain do not display the same invariability. On the contrary, how people respond to events depends on when and where they occur, who is present, and what the individuals hope to accomplish. (p. 54)

Thus, the "bad rep" that theory often gets in public health and health promotion may indeed be the product of public health's insistence in approaching human behavior as resulting from fixed, universal forces. Negative views of theory may be in place because we insist in asking the wrong questions because we fail to admit that health behaviors lie in the domain of praxis-type experience and, therefore, lead to practical reasoning, or phronesis-type knowledge, not episteme-type knowledge. Current theories of health behavior provide one size fits all answers to questions such as "what causes people to choose a healthy lifestyle?" or "what may lead people to better manage their diets and eating habits?" Most of the answers we now have tend to be "universal," fixed, blatantly ignoring that health behaviors are context-bound and contingent on their socio-cultural-economic contexts.

If this might indeed be the case, then why would we expect practitioners to *want* to use these theories when they really don't answer the right-here-right-now questions practitioners have? For example, if a health educator wonders, "How can I help Ms. Smith manage her diabetes, given the small retirement income she manages and the large family she always says 'comes first'?" then the answers provided by health behavior theories such as "increase Ms. Smith's self-efficacy" (Bandura, 1997) and "increase her perception of the severity of diabetes" (Champion & Skinner, 2008) are totally irrelevant. Actually, if the health educator is not careful, focusing on these "scientific" answers can do more harm than good (or become iatrogenic—more about this in Chapter 8): Because Ms. Smith's context (low income, large family, and her place within this family network) seems to shape her health problems, intervention attempts to increase self-efficacy or perceived severity of the disease may only contribute to enhancing Ms. Smith's anxiety and guilt (Becker, 1993). The practitioner's intervention—if he or she is concerned about applying one size fits all health behavior theories to develop her educational program—may transform Ms. Smith from a "person at risk" into an "anxious person at risk" contributing to exacerbate what has been dubbed an "epidemic of apprehension" (Becker, 1993, p. 2).

From this perspective, you might even conclude it may, in fact, be positive for theory and practice to maintain a healthy distance in public health. Yet, I would argue that the current status of theory and practice in public health (this ambivalent, love–hate relationship you see described in more detail in Chapter 3) is a significant symptom of an underlying illness we have institutionalized in our profession.

To separate theory and praxis (or theoretical thinking from action) is an artifact. There is nothing more valuable, more enlightening, and more empowering than the marriage of the right type of question with the appropriate answer, to build understanding, to shape professional practice, and to sharpen our professional awareness. This is another important point in this chapter, so take note: Theoretical thinking that is relevant is intricately tied to practice. Divorcing the two becomes nonsense (no sense). It is breaking something that is a unit, a "one," a whole, into pieces and expecting the pieces to survive and perform on their own—like splitting a peanut butter and jelly sandwich by pulling apart the slices of bread. Try doing this, and you have nothing: not a peanut butter and jelly sandwich, not peanut butter and bread, not bread and jelly. If split, the final product is something else, but it isn't a peanut butter and jelly sandwich anymore!

Paulo Freire—the Brazilian critical theorist and philosopher of education whom health promoters have come to know well due to his contributions related to empowerment theories (Wallerstein, Sanchez-Merki, & Dow, 1997)—has articulated this unity between theory and practice appropriately. For him, the relationship is the same as the one between action and reflection. He calls the relationship between theory and practice a dialogical one. For Freire, our individual behavior and the way we live in society represent a constant "conversation" or "dialogue" between our doing and our thinking about what was done—the thinking about what was done, in turn, shaping what will be done next, and so forth in a continual iterative process.

John Willinsky (1998), writing about theory in the context of teaching literature, argues this point quite eloquently:

> Try thinking of how we practice theory, that is, of how theory is a form of practice. After all, theory is practiced, whether by a young child facing a plate full of different foods or a teacher in front of a class on the first day. Theory takes practice. Theory shapes practice.

> Take this a step further and consider how this habit of naming one thing as "practice" and another as "theory" is in itself the work or practice of theory. It is a theoretical distinction. Such is the practice of theory. In this way, it seems fair to say that a theory of the world is what enables us to work with it. Or to put this another way, the world makes little sense without a theory about it. Our practices exist by virtue of our theories. (p. 244)

When relevant questions and appropriate answers are developed and applied, what you have is theory and practice as action and reflection, or reflexive praxis: two sides of the same coin. If you have an inclination for metaphysical images, think of this unity as being similar to you: You consist of a physical dimension (your body) and a nonphysical dimension (your soul, your mind, or whatever is you that is not solely physical). If we were to try to separate these two dimensions of yourself, what would happen? Pretty disastrous, wouldn't you say? And so it is when trying to artificially separate theory from practice and action from reflection. No wonder health-promotion professionals (and students) complain that theory is dry, irrelevant, and boring. People would complain that you were dry and boring too if only your dead body walked around, interacting with others, with no personality, emotions, hopes, dreams and quirks. Your beauty lies in the dynamic life force within you, the interaction among all the dimensions that constitute you!

If we think about theorizing as the interplay, the "dance" or the constant dialogue between a specific type of question and its respective answers, when the questions asked and the answers given match and when both emerge from action, theory/theoretical thinking and practice are one. This constant, dynamic dance/dialogue of action and reflection, theory and practice, to me makes the two inseparable. It also reinforces the notion that theory (or theorizing) is itself a type of practice. If you remember what we said before, regarding what it is that theory *does*, you will conclude that because theory questions actions, questions the status quo (the manner in which we do things), seeks the most plausible and meaningful answers, and builds a narrative in which to frame the questions and the answers, it is indeed engaged in quite a bit of practical tasks! It does a lot!

In this way, theory has a necessary practical dimension; without practice (understood as everyday living), theory wouldn't happen—it wouldn't exist. Conversely, without theory, living would be undefined and meaningless, merely biological subsistence. Therefore, to divorce theory from practice (which is, in fact, what you will observe when you look at much of the current public health practice) becomes detrimental to our sense making: neither can we explain our practice and those things that are extremely relevant to us nor can we improve our way of doing things because we don't question them.

FINAL THOUGHTS

I would like to add one final observation regarding scientific theories' claims to their ability to *predict* behaviors. Despite widespread dissatisfaction in our field with health behavior theories' power to describe, foretell, and therefore, prevent risky behaviors, the mere notion that theories aspire to predict behavior with precision and efficiency is, to me, very scary.

Imagine this scenario: a certain theory proposes that an individual's theoretical self-esteem (TSE—defined as the regard one has for one's self in terms of the ability to think theoretically) is associated with his or her theorizing behavior. If I—the theorizing expert—knew the TSE scores of a certain group of students, for instance, I could easily predict to what extent those students practice theorizing behaviors, or better yet, I could devise educational or marketing strategies to enhance that group's TSE and thus to get more frequent theorizing behavior out of them! Thank goodness there's no such thing as TSE (interestingly enough, though, there is such a thing as "web-esteem"—so it may not be long till we see TSE as a bona-fide theoretical construct; see Brock, 2006).

While the construct of TSE is merely a product of my imagination and predictions of ability to think theoretically are not life threatening, the ability to predict behavior is not science fiction. It is, in fact, one of the main goals of scientific theorizing, and as we have learned from the natural sciences, it can be done. *Should* it be done, however?[1] Buchanan, for instance, argues that if our health behavior theories and our health promotion methods were to become ultraefficient at predicting and changing health behaviors, our autonomy as human beings would be lost:

Buchanan (2004) writes:

> To me, the quest to find such power is deeply disturbing. Whoever controlled these new behavioral technologies would have the power to control your and my behavior. If effective scientific models [or theories] were ever developed, then the government, for example, would have the power to decide whether I would eat that dessert, exercise today, smoke pot, have sex outside marriage, or change any other behavior that it wanted to control. If effective scientific models were ever developed, then the very foundations of human autonomy, responsibility, dignity, and respect would be destroyed. We would have no autonomy, no moral responsibility, and no dignity because (1) scientists would have identified the causes of the behavior in question, and ipso facto, (2) they would have the power

---

[1]Notice the theorizing attempt here to question the status quo regarding how we use behavioral theories in health promotion. In this case, it took a simple question: Should scientists be able to predict human behavior efficiently?

to change or eliminate that behavior. It would, in short, be a brave new world, beyond freedom and dignity. (p. 150)

Granted: Theorists and researchers are quick to say prediction is not very precise at the level of the individual, therefore, I really can't do a good job of anticipating your theorizing behavior (what a relief!). Prediction works best at the level of aggregate data—when dealing with averages—and with populations or groups, not with individual persons. Even so, if you think that public policy usually predicates upon such "averages" and upon target groups and/or populations, it can still be a scary thought that we would try to predict (and, therefore, control and tweak) people's behaviors.

Well, this is enough for now on the problematic implications of using scientific health behavior theories efficiently to promote behavior change. There is more on this in other sections of the book.

In concluding, I believe you have rarely been challenged to think about theory this broadly. When was the last time you read something proposing that theory might be beautiful? Well, it is, and my goal is to walk you through the various manifestations of theory, to introduce you to its most attractive (and nonattractive) features, and to guide you to refine your theoretical thinking skills. I trust you will, after reading this book, invest in your own theoretical thinking and evaluate the current status of theorizing within public health. Oh, yes, I do want to offer you guidelines for using scientific theories in research and in practice because to use health behavior theories this way is still the bread-and-butter of public health. I hope, however, that "using" theory becomes, in your professional worldview, only one way to approach theoretical thinking about health. My goal is for you to feel challenged to take a stab at theorizing, to know you can become more than just a "theory consumer" or a "theory applicator" (I know, it sounds like a makeup tool; horrible term!), and to seriously consider becoming a "theorizer" or a theorist. In a sense, this book is about theories (some would say a "meta-theory" text), but it is about more than theory, too: It's about you, your approach to theory, research, and practice, as well as your discovering the exciting places where theoretical thinking can take *you*.

Theory is a basic survival skill. This may surprise those who believe it to be a special activity of experts of a certain kind. True, there are professional . . . theorists, usually academics. But this fact does not exclude my belief that . . . theory is something done necessarily, and often well, by people with no particular professional credential. When it is done well, by whomever, it can be a source of uncommon pleasure. (Lemert, 1993, p. 1)

SUGGESTIONS FOR PRACTICING THEORETICAL THINKING

1. Conduct an informal survey of your colleagues. Ask them this: "When I say the word 'theory' (or the phrase 'health behavior theories'), what comes to mind?" Assess whether their answers carry positive, negative, or neutral connotations.

2. Ask yourself how is the term "theory" being used in health education and public health? You could write a systematic literature review of the topic and submit your findings for publication.

3. Promote a panel discussion regarding (1) what types of ideas have earned the label of "theory" in health education and public health and (2) whether public health is, indeed, asking the appropriate theoretical questions regarding health promotion (i.e., whether we should focus so much in finding invariable, universal causes for human behavior). Invite a group of faculty and students in your school to debate the issue and/or begin a brown-bag lunch series to revisit the questions periodically.

4. Familiarize yourself with David Buchanan's work and his critical analysis of health education/health promotion. Figure out where you stand vis-à-vis his critique of our practice.

5. Learn more about Paulo Freire's vision of education as dialogical or something that happens in dialogue between teachers and learners. You may find some interesting (and inspiring ideas) for your own work in public health!

REFERENCES

Bandura, A. (1997). *Self-Efficacy: The Exercise of Control.* New York: W.H. Freeman and Company.

Becker, M. H. (1993). A medical sociologist looks at health promotion. *Journal of Health and Social Behavior, 34*(1), 1–6.

Brock, R. (2006, July 21). Women diminish their web-surfing skills, but the sexes are even study finds. *The Chronicle of Higher Education.*

Buchanan, D. R. (2000). *An Ethic for Health Promotion: Rethinking the Sources of Human Well-Being.* New York: Oxford University Press. By permission of Oxford University Press.

Buchanan, D. R. (2004). Two models for defining the relationship between theory and practice in nutrition education: is the scientific method meeting our needs? *Journal of Nutrition Education and Behavior, 36,* 146–154.

Champion, V. L., & Skinner, C. S. (2008). The health belief model. In K. Glanz, B. K. Rimer, & K. Viswanath (Eds.), *Health Behavior and Health Education: Theory, Research, and Practice* (4th ed., pp. 45–65). San Francisco: Jossey-Bass.

Chen, H.-T. (1990). *Theory-Driven Evaluations.* Newbury Park, CA: Sage Publications.

Cohen, B. P. (1980). *Developing Sociological Knowledge: Theory and Method.* Englewood Cliffs, NJ: Prentice-Hall.

Denzin, N. K. (1970). *The Research Act: A Theoretical Introduction to Sociological Methods.* Chicago: Aldine Publishing Company.

DiClemente, R. J., Crosby, R. A., & Kegler, M. C. (Eds.). (2002). *Emerging Theories in Health Promotion Practice and Research: Strategies for Improving Public Health.* San Francisco: Jossey-Bass.

Edberg, M. (2007). *Social and Behavioral Theory in Public Health.* Sudbury, MA: Jones and Bartlett.

Frank, A. W. (1995). *The Wounded Storyteller: Body, Illness, and Ethics.* Chicago: The University of Chicago Press.

Glanz, K., Rimer, B. K., & Viswanath, K. (2008). *Health Behavior and Health Education: Theory, Research, and Practice* (4th ed.). San Francisco: Jossey-Bass.

Hoffmann, R. (2003). Why buy that theory? *American Scientist, 91,* 9–11.

Kurtz, M. L. (2006). *The JFK Assassination Debates: Lone Gunman versus Conspiracy.* Lawrence, KA: University Press of Kansas.

Lemert, C. (1993). *Social Theory: The Multicultural and Classic Readings.* Boulder, CO: Westview Press.

Lewin, K. (1951). *Field Theory in Social Science: Selected Theoretical Papers.* New York: Harper & Brothers Publishers.

Nash, R. J. (2004). *Liberating Scholarly Writing: The Power of Personal Narrative.* New York: Teachers College Press.

Nealon, J., & Giroux, S. S. (2003). *The Theory Toolbox: Critical Concepts for the Humanities, Arts, and Social Sciences.* New York: Rowman & Littlefield Publishers.

Pedhazur, E. J., & Schmelkin, L. P. (1991). Theories, problems, and hypotheses. In E. Pedhazur & L. P. Schmelkin (Eds.), *Measurement, Design and Analysis: An Integrated Approach* (pp. 180–210). Hillsdale, NJ: Lawrence Erlbaum Associates Publishers.

Schwandt, T. A. (2001). *Dictionary of Qualitative Inquiry* (2nd ed.). Thousand Oaks, CA: Sage Publications.

Turner, J. H. (1986). *The Structure of Sociological Theory.* Chicago: The Dorsey Press.

Wallerstein, N., Sanchez-Merki, V., & Dow, L. (1997). Feirian praxis in health education and community organizing: a case study of an adolescent prevention program. In M. Minkler (Ed.), *Community Organizing & Community Building for Health* (pp. 195–211). New Brunswick, NJ: Rutgers University Press.

Willinsky, J. (1998). Teaching literature is teaching in theory. *Theory Into Practice, 37*(3), 244–250.

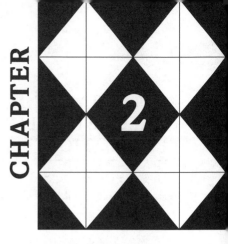

CHAPTER 2

Why Think Theoretically About Health Promotion?

Learning Objectives

When you finish reading this chapter, you will be able to:

1. Offer a coherent rationale for why we should think theoretically about health promotion.
2. Explain why thinking theoretically about health promotion forms the basis for social justice and ethical practice.
3. Identify professional responsibilities of public health workers, related to theoretical thinking.
4. Recognize the theoretical thinking efforts currently underway in public health.
5. Recall how theoretical thinking guides research efforts in public health.

RATIONALE FOR THINKING THEORETICALLY ABOUT HEALTH PROMOTION

Hoping I was able to clarify the concept of theoretical thinking in the previous chapter, I now would like to answer a couple of questions you may have asked all along:

> Why should we think theoretically about health promotion?
> Isn't observing and collecting data related to public health issues and practice, enough?

The simple and immediate answer to the latter question is "no, not enough." The not-so-simple and more elaborate answers to the former questions are discussed later. As you read, please keep in mind a couple of points: first, the reasons for thinking theoretically I discuss in this chapter are presented individually, in a quasi-disconnected fashion. In practice, however, all of these reasons correlate and interact synergistically. I present them individually, for didactic purposes only. Second, there are other reasons for thinking theoretically besides the ones I propose here. The seven reasons described in this chapter represent, therefore, my own personal bias and worldview, shaped by the thinking of many scholars in public health and other disciplines. I challenge you to think of other (your own) reasons for thinking theoretically about health promotion and to consistently engage in this type of thinking throughout your professional career.

Reason 1: Because Theoretical Thinking Infuses Ethics and Social Justice into Public Health Practice[1]

It lasted 40 years: from 1932 to 1972. It was characterized as one of the most infamous man-made tragedies in the history of American science. Its legacy tainted

---

[1] I define practice, here, as more than planning, implementation, and evaluation of health promoting interventions. For the purposes of this chapter, practice is defined as Fee and Brown (2000) characterized it:

> First, "practice" as "praxis" means the total framework of one's professional life, including the ideology or worldview that guides one's actions, the framework of values used to set priorities, the commitment to translate these values and ideas into daily activities, and the expectation that by doing so consistently, one can transform the world in which one lives. Second, "practice," in the sense of "vocation," means acting according to a sense of calling or mission" (p. 690).

medical- and community-based research efforts long into the 21st century (Freimuth et al., 2001). It became known as The Tuskegee Study. Its purpose was

> . . . to determine the long-term course of [syphilis] in the absence of treatment and to note the peculiarities of the disease in black men. (There was widespread, mistaken belief among physicians that blacks responded differently to the disease than did whites). (Garrett, 2000, p. 321)

The study was conducted among a group of 600 black men (399 cases and 201 controls) in Macon County, Alabama. In 1932, Macon County exhibited one of the highest syphilis rates in the world (Garrett, 2000; Jones, 1993). Medical and public health researchers saw Macon County as a natural laboratory at their disposal. The Tuskegee Institute (since 1985, Tuskegee University), "founded by Booker T. Washington to educate freed slaves and their descendents," was housed in that county. Because the Tuskegee Institute relied heavily on federal funding, participation in the syphilis study became an opportunity for the institute to partner with the government and obtain much-needed revenue. The institute volunteered to contribute to the study by donating office space, hospital facilities, and laboratory resources (Hunter-Gault, 1997; Tuskegee University, 2008).

If the racist assumptions underlying its purpose weren't reason enough, the study became a hallmark of unethical medical research because it relied, intentionally, on deceiving participants and later, when treatment for syphilis became available, on withholding the treatment from those who were already ill:

> In order to lure men into the study, none of the patients was told he had syphilis—rather, they learned from the Tuskegee staff that they suffered from "bad blood. . . ." Initially imagined as a six-month study, the Tuskegee experiment would last until 1972. In all that time, the Macon County men and their families would never be told that they had syphilis. Nor were they provided with penicillin in 1943 when USPHS [United States Public Health Service] researchers discovered that it could cure syphilis. (Garrett, 2000, pp. 321–322)

Sixty-five years after the study began—on May 16, 1997—President Bill Clinton apologized, in the name of the United States Government, to the handful of survivors and their families gathered at the White House for the historical event. Addressing the survivors, the President stated: "The people who ran the study at Tuskegee diminished the stature of man [sic] by abandoning the most basic ethical precepts. They forgot their pledge to heal and repair." (Hunter-Gault, 1997)

To this day, the after-shocks of the study reverberate in the scientific and medical communities. Survey findings suggest that knowledge of (or, more precisely, misconceptions about) the study may negatively impact people's willingness to participate in medical research (Freimuth et al., 2001; Garrett, 2000; Katz,

Kegeles, & Kressin 2006; McCallum, Arekere, Green, Katz, & Rivers, 2006). Conversely, modern-day efforts to protect human subjects who take part in research—through institutional review boards' approval of study protocols—have become tangible corrective measures resulting from the Tuskegee debacle (Flicker, Travers, Guta, McDonald, & Meagher, 2007; Oakes, 2002).

Especially because we now live in an era that strongly emphasizes protection for people and animals taking part in research studies, we can't help but ask, "How could something like the Tuskegee Study ever happen?" In a competent attempt to explain how, in the book *Bad Blood*, James Jones weaves countless pieces of information, connects a myriad of characters entering and exiting the Tuskegee scene over the years, and describes in lengthy details the study's background (historical, social, economic, and scientific). Moreover, he carefully builds the plot that culminates with the unveiling, to the general public, of the study's continued existence: On July 25, 1972, a story authored by journalist Jean Heller appears in the *Washington Star*. Only then, does the U.S. society learn of the ordeal of the study's participants (Jones, 1993).

While reading Jones' book, I probably reacted as the typical reader who couldn't stop asking—despite the carefully woven narrative—"how on earth?" Because the history of the study is extremely complex and drawn out, I had a hard time connecting the many dots that Jones offered and failed to construct a simplified picture of the underlying motives. A single section in the book, however, brought home to me the basic, fundamental reason for Tuskegee having happened and having prevailed for so long. In that section, Jones critically discusses the system of peer review in the field of medicine in place in the 1930s. Those were times when codes of ethics outlining the protection of human subjects in research were nonexistent. The atrocities of Nazi experiments with humans had yet to occur, and physicians were gravely concerned with "preserving professional autonomy," not with defining "good practice" (Jones, 1993, p. 96). For me, the "aha!" moment came packaged in a single phrase in that section:

> Perhaps, too, the problem of defining with any degree of exactitude what constituted "sound medical practice" [during the 1930s] simply staggered a profession [medicine] largely composed of technicians and almost wholly composed of *people uninterested in theorizing*. (Jones, 1993, p. 96, emphasis mine)

With this sentence, I was able to finally put my finger on the root of the problem: Tuskegee didn't happen because scientists conducting the study *abandoned* basic ethical precepts, as former President Clinton stated in his apology speech (and I do hate to disagree with a former president). It happened because medical doctors, during that historical moment, were trained to become healing technicians, versed on methods, strategies, and procedures for treatment and cure. They were not being trained to inquire, to question the status quo (why are we doing this?), to reflect on their practice. Their training had failed to foster the habit of theoretical thinking, of theorizing. The same argument applies to the public health workforce at the time. In the spirit of a good Nike advertisement to be developed nearly a half a century later, they just "did it."

From my perspective, there has never been an account as powerful as this one, to drive home the point that without the work of theory, professional ethics might as well be thrown out the window. No theory, no ethics. No theorizing, no reflection upon practice. No dialogue between theory and practice, no learning, no respect, no justice. It's that simple.

Theorizing—because it questions the status quo, and promotes reflection about practice and research—facilitates the groundwork for ethics and promotion of social justice within any profession, but especially within public health (Marmede, Schmidt, & Rikers, 2007). According to Fee and Brown (2000), "If the ideal of justice is abandoned by public health insiders, we have lost the very purpose of our mission" (p. 690).

Whenever someone asks you about the importance of theoretical thinking in health promotion, tell your listener the Tuskegee Study story and emphasize this point: The medical establishment's complete disinterest in theorizing, in questioning the status quo, in reflecting about its practice created a technique-oriented monster of a profession, concerned exclusively with itself. This is clearly a case where ignoring the practice of theory, far from being harmless, had horrendous consequences.

Reason 2: Because Theoretical Thinking Represents a Moral Duty and a Professional Responsibility

Another reason for thinking theoretically, also in the realm of ethics, is this: it's a duty, a professional responsibility. But what does professional responsibility mean?

Professionals of all types have certain tasks they must carry out in their daily practice, as well as values they must continually uphold; together, tasks and values constitute professional responsibilities. These professionals are held accountable for these responsibilities by their colleagues and their clients (and by society, as a whole). In other words, if a professional does not abide by commonly shared codes of conduct and professional standards, he/she is subject to sanctions, reprimands, or punishment; if, in contrast, that professional follows all guidelines and rules of conduct, he/she is worthy of praise and merit.

This notion of professional responsibility, as a set of tasks, procedures, or moral principles that should be followed, is not difficult to grasp; after all, most professions have certain codes of conduct or ethics and guidelines for their professional practice. It might be, however, a bit more difficult to "see" theoretical thinking as one of these professional responsibilities. Why would theorizing be a duty, a responsibility?

In the book *The Wounded Storyteller,* the author argues that ill people have a responsibility to tell their stories, to theorize about their experience. For him,

> Ill people's storytelling is informed by a sense of *responsibility to the commonsense world* [emphasis mine] and represents one way of living *for* the other. People tell stories not just to work out their own changing identities [when struck with illness], but also to guide others who will follow them. They seek not to provide a map that can guide others—each must create his own—but rather to witness the experience of reconstructing one's own map. Witnessing is one duty to the commonsensical and to others." (Frank, 1995, p. 17)

If we agree with Frank that there is a sense of duty in telling our stories about health and illness and if we believe theorizing is a process of making sense of health and illness through storytelling, then, by extension, theorizing is a duty. Theorizing or attributing meaning to our professional reality becomes a responsibility to both the commonsense world and our professional world.

To me, this is a very compelling reason for investing in theoretical thinking in health promotion: We owe it to the public, to our clients. We owe them not merely the development of efficient and effective tools and strategies to promote health. We owe them the responsibility to reflect on our practice continually, question our methods, reform our views, and construct the narratives that give them meaning. At the same time, we have the responsibility of witnessing our clients' own narratives, their attempts of making meaning of their lives, and their contributions to our own understanding of health and illness (Alderson, 1998; Biswas et al., 2007; Hinyard & Kreuter, 2007).

Please don't think I'm romanticizing about some pie-in-the-sky, idealized way of practicing health promotion when I bring up this "duty" argument. I haven't made this up. Theorizing is, indeed, a behavior embedded in six of the seven areas of professional responsibility for health educators, defined by the National Commission for Health Education Credentialing (the organization responsible for certifying professional health educators, nationwide; see www.nchec.org) (Gilmore, Olsen, Taub, & Connell, 2005). For instance, as part of Area I—Assess Individual and Community Needs for Health Education—subcompetency C refers to identifying "diverse factors that influence health behaviors" (i.e., theorizing about cause-and-effect relationships), and subcompetency E consists of identifying "factors that foster or hinder the process of health education" (i.e., theorizing about sociopolitical contexts) (National Commission for Health Education Credentialing). As another example, embedded in Area VII—Communicate and Advocate for Health and Health Education—we find further references to the professional duty of theorizing and attributing meaning to health promotion practice, even though the terms "theoretical thinking" or "theory" do not appear in the wording: "Competency A—*Analyze and respond to current and future needs in health education.* Sub-Competency: Analyze factors (e.g., social, cultural, demographic, political) that influence decision makers (National Commission for Health Education Credentialing)."

Analyzing health education needs and factors that influence decision makers are all theoretical tasks. They require understanding of multiple levels of cause-and-effect relationships, knowledge of current social science and political science theories, as well as the development of a narrative/logical structure through which they can be communicated.

One example of this type of theoretical thinking is an article I co-authored with one of my now-former doctoral students, Lei-Shih Chen. In this article, titled "Entering the Public Health Genomics Era: Why Must Health Educators Develop Genomic Competencies?" we propose and develop five arguments supporting the notion that health educators must begin to think about developing their genomic competencies. We begin by defining genetics, genomics, public health genetics, public health genomics, and genomic competencies. We then provide the five arguments and carefully develop each one, based on information available to public health professionals at the time of the writing. The five arguments are as follows (Chen & Goodson, 2007):

Argument 1—Because leading professional organizations have advocated the incorporation of genomics into health promotion practice.

Argument 2—Because health educators' professional competencies and responsibilities encourage and corroborate the incorporation of genomics into health promotion practice.

Argument 3—Because health educators' genomic competencies can significantly impact the lay public's utilization of and satisfaction with public health genetics/genomic services.

Argument 4—Because by developing their genomic competencies, health educators are better able to meet emerging health needs.

Argument 5—Because genomics and public health are generating unique opportunities for interdisciplinary collaboration, research funding, and employment.

If you read through the article, you will find that Chen's and my task, as authors, was not to report on research findings or document an experiment of any kind. The work we did was purely theoretical: It involved identifying factors and existing elements that could be connected through logic and presented to readers in a persuasive fashion. Given the historical moment health promotion finds itself embedded in, Chen and I felt we had a professional obligation to alert the field to the current and future need for health education to begin incorporating genomic competencies, to help the workforce think through these needs, and to devise mechanisms to address them.

So…not only do we have a duty to tell stories that make sense of realities in the commonsense world, we also have a responsibility to our professional world of seeking out meaning, reflecting about practice, and making sense of health promotion, health threats, and illnesses. Theoretical thinking, as we have seen, is the essential tool for meeting such responsibilities and, as professionals, we are accountable for employing that tool.

Reason 3: Because Theoretical Thinking Guides the Profession

As you have just read, among health educators' professional areas of responsibility listed by NCHEC, we find this: advocating for, and promoting, health education as a profession (Area VII). Whether we choose to consider health education, in particular, or any other dimension of public health, more broadly, makes little difference. Within all of public health's dimensions, thinking theoretically about the field, its direction, goals, and values is an essential task for grounding and steadying the profession within the parameters of ethics, social justice, and effectiveness.

Not many scholars in public health and health education have dedicated their scholarship to thinking theoretically about the professional dimensions of health promotion. Those committed to the task have, no doubt, shaped and directed the field, leading all of us to more effective and ethical practice. (For a brief historical review of important theoretical contributions to public health practice, see Green, 2006.)

When thinking about those who have, indeed, shaped the field from a theoretical perspective, I'm reminded particularly of Lawrence W. Green and Marshall W. Kreuter's work, developing and refining the PRECEDE–PROCEED model. Even though not a scientific theory, per se, the model resulted from careful theoretical thinking and attempts to make intervention planning logical, theory-based, and user-friendly (Green & Kreuter, 2005). Along the same lines of contributing toward planning and practice through the development of in-depth planning models,

I think of the work of L. Kay Bartholomew, Guy Parcel, Gerjo Kok, and Nell H. Gottlieb (my mentor during doctoral studies' days) in developing Intervention Mapping. Intervention Mapping is a strategy that facilitates effective decision making, at each and every step in the planning, implementation and evaluation of a health promotion intervention. The strategy makes it easier for practitioners to identify "a set of well-defined antecedents or determinants of behavior and environmental conditions" to target in their interventions, thus ensuring that their efforts are more likely to be effective (Bartholomew, Parcel, Kok, & Gottlieb, 2006, p. 4).

Among the handful of theoretical thinkers in our field, I'm also reminded of the work carried out by Meredith Minkler questioning the status of health promotion and the paths chosen by the profession (Minkler, 1999; Robertson & Minkler, 1994). For instance, in an article titled, "Health Education, Health Promotion and the Open Society: An Historical Perspective" (published in 1989, this article has now become a "classic" in the field), Minkler examines the historical development of two alternative directions health promotion began to face in the 1980s: "the first focusing primarily on personal behavior change and the [second] on a broad empowerment/environmental model of health promotion" (Minkler, 1989, p. 17). In that article, Minkler provides an outstanding example of theoretical thinking: She revisits some of the questioning that had taken place in the late 60s regarding the direction health promotion might be taking, warns the field of potential inherent dangers, and poses historical arguments to make her point clear. Here are the first few paragraphs of that article. As you may notice, it's difficult to believe she wrote this 20 years ago and not yesterday.

> Twenty years ago, health education leader Dorothy Nyswander[2] reflected back upon her career, measuring her work and the work of her profession, against the criteria of an open society. She defined the latter as a society that concerns itself

---

[2] Dorothy Bird Nyswander was considered the "mother of health education." One of the founders of the School of Public Health at the University of California at Berkeley, she was actively engaged in public health work for more than 60 years. Nyswander (1967) believed and promoted the concept of an "Open Society," one where

> justice is the same for every man; where dissent is taken seriously as an index of something wrong or something needed; where diversity is respected; where pressure groups cannot stifle and control the will of the majority or castigate the individual; where education brings upward mobility to all; where the best of health care is available to all; where poverty is a community disgrace not an individual's weakness; where greed for possessions and success is replaced by inner fire for excellence and honor; where desires for power *over* men become satisfactions with the use of power *for* men. (p. 11)

with the rights and dignity of the individual, respect for diversity and dissent and with increasing social justice and individual sense of control and self-determination.

While making clear her pride in health education's accomplishments, Dr. Nyswander also expressed concern over its limitations. She went on to admonish health educators to *redefine and significantly broaden their professional goals*, bringing them into closer alignment with the goals of an open society [emphasis mine].

Two decades later [1980s], health educators are again being asked—by sources ranging from private hospitals to the World Health Organization—*to reexamine their professional roles and to make some dramatic shifts* [emphasis mine]. This time around, however, we face two quite contradictory proscriptions for change. And to make matters even more confusing, both are being put forward under the rubric of health promotion. Which direction we choose will have tremendous implications for the future of the field—and more important, for the contributions that health educators may make toward improving the public's health. (Minkler, 1989, pp. 17–18)

In recent years, Minkler's writing has focused on developing logical arguments buttressing the importance, methods, and implications of community-based participatory research (CBPR) in public health (Minkler, 2000; Minkler & Wallerstein, 2003; Minkler, Blackwell, Thompson, & Tamir, 2003). Defined as "a collaborative process that equitably involves all partners in the research process and recognizes the unique strengths that each brings" (Minkler et al., 2003, p. 1211), CBPR has been touted by health scholars, governments, private and philanthropic organizations, as a more desirable form of research and problem-solving action strategy within communities (Minkler, 2004). Nevertheless, CBPR presents its share of challenges and difficulties, and Minkler exercises her responsibility to her profession, pointing out the challenges and offering compelling recommendations (Minkler, 2004).

Among the theoretical thinkers who have helped to shape health promotion, I also think of those who have contributed to developing and applying health behavior theories, such as the editors and the authors of the textbooks *Health Behavior and Health Education: Theory, Research, and Practice* and *Emerging Theories in Health Promotion Practice and Research* (Glanz, Rimer, & Viswanath, 2008; DiClemente, Crosby, & Kegler, 2002). Among the scholars dedicating their careers to developing and testing health behavior theories, I especially recall those who first promoted a systems-thinking approach to health promotion, through the use of an ecological framework (McLeroy, Bibeau, Steckler, & Glanz, 1988; Simons-Morton, Simons-Morton, Parcel, & Bunker, 1988). The ecological framework highlighted the need to go beyond individual-level factors to explain health behavior and include interpersonal, community, and policy elements as well. Introducing the notion of multilevel influences on individuals' health behavior represented a paradigm shift, or one of those "tipping point" moments, when an entire field sees itself confronted with new information, new ways of thinking (Gladwell, 2000; Rogers, 1962).

More recently, I also think of the scholars who have advanced the application of systems theory[3] to understanding human health (Green, 2006; Homer & Hirsch, 2006; Leischow & Milstein, 2006; Resnicow & Page, 2008; Trochim, Cabrera, Milstein, Gallagher, & Leischow, 2006). Systems science, while including ecological perspectives, goes beyond these models to include advances "in fields such as system dynamics and complexity theory" (Trochim et al., 2006, p. 538). Such new ways of thinking often preclude looking back: After we understood the importance and the force of ecological influences, it was nearly impossible to continue to think about health behaviors as shaped merely by personal or individual-level factors. As we begin to approach public health as a complex adaptive system, it becomes increasingly difficult to focus exclusively on individual elements of this system (e.g., local health departments), in isolation from the entire network of public health services.

In recent years, I find David R. Buchanan's writings constitute an important theoretical reflection about our profession. At the time of this writing, Buchanan is a Full Professor of Community Health Education at the School of Public Health and Health Sciences at the University of Massachusetts. He has authored numerous journal articles, but I find his book *An Ethic for Health Promotion* one of the most important contributions of his career. His perspective has significantly impacted my thinking, as he pointedly raises the difficult questions about the direction health education, specifically, and public health in general, has taken (Buchanan, 1994, 1998, 2000, 2004, 2006b, 2008).

As Buchanan sees it, health promotion has abandoned its education and humanities roots in favor of privileging the ideology of the natural sciences. Motivated perhaps by the need to compete for federal funding, to demonstrate effectiveness (to show that health interventions "work"), and to garner admiration or prestige, the field has touted the use of scientific methods

---

[3] The term "Systems Theory" refers to "an approach or perspective in several disciplines that emphasizes studying the interrelations of the parts of a whole (the system) more than studying components in isolation from their position in an organization" (Vogt, 2005, p. 230).

(including scientific theories of health behavior) to control and manage people's risk or health-promoting behaviors. Yet, as he strategically points out, our record of success using such methods has not been impressive. Here's an example of how physicians view our "scientific" attempts (Chehab, Pfeffer, Vargas, Chen, & Irigoyen, 2007):

> The prevalence of American adolescent obesity tripled in the past 30 years; currently over 17% of adolescents are obese. Most childhood obesity interventions are rooted in theories of social learning and the health belief model, and focus on enhancing health education, physical education, and food within the school environment. In a review of recent programs, only [three] American interventions significantly impacted weight. . . . Given the limited success of most childhood obesity interventions, alternate approaches need to be explored. (p. 474)

Not a very flattering compliment to our efforts, I would say. Yet Buchanan has emphasized the need to consider criticism such as this seriously and to honestly re-examine the course health promotion has chosen. In a reply to an editorial in the journal *Health Education & Behavior*, Buchanan (2006a) stated,

> There are moments when I despair about the state of our profession. . . . We have made a colossal categorical mistake. We have foolishly and egregiously applied the standards of scientific success to what is intrinsically a moral and political enterprise: deliberating about how to live well. The value of health education lies in promoting ethical principles regarding human well-being and quality of life, social justice, human autonomy, and responsibility, not technologies of behavior control. (p. 308)

Why so few health promotion scholars engage in this type of theoretical thinking about the profession is understandable: to think this way is disquieting and disturbing (Willinsky, 1998, p. 245). It rattles the status quo cage and ruffles many feathers in the process (my apologies for the double metaphor!) As Willinsky (1998, p. 249) describes when addressing this type of theorizing in the field of education, "The encounter with theory leaves [us] aware of *theory's work of disrupting and unsettling, exposing and revealing* desires that may be, once known, dangerous in practice and not just in theory [emphasis mine]."

Yet, isn't this the work of theory after all? To disrupt, unsettle, expose, and reveal? Without such labor, the practice of health promotion is doomed to meaninglessness or, worse yet, to other fields imposing *their* meanings upon on our work. I make this latter point clearer in Reason # 4. Read on.

Reason 4: Because Theoretical Thinking Prevents Ideological Takeover, or Hegemony

You are probably familiar with the terms *ideology* and *hegemony*. A set of rather complex constructs, their definitions have been refined many times throughout the history of Western thought. For now, however, let's define ideology and hegemony in their simplest terms. Ideology represents the "integrated assertions, theories and aims that constitute a sociopolitical program" (Merriam-Webster). The phrase "sociopolitical program" here does not mean a degree in political science. It means the collection of plans societies have for governing themselves, for administering all that goes on in their midst. In turn, hegemony happens when one social group's ideology dominates another group and becomes the predominant influence over this group—in other words, an ideology takeover.

Now, here's my argument: if public health ideology—or the assertions, theories, and aims that define public health—is not being construed and shaped by the public health workforce itself, then another ideology—developed by professionals outside the field—will fill the void. Public health practice cannot exist without an ideology (or set of theories) to frame it, to give it meaning. But who articulates that meaning? Who builds the public health narratives that guide the field? The meanings and the ideology will be constructed—one way or another—because human beings have a need to attribute meaning to their actions. Who conceives this ideology becomes then an interesting and nontrivial matter to consider: If not we, public health professionals, then who? If we're not theorizing, either because we don't know how or don't want to bother, other professionals (psychologists, sociologists, anthropologists, ethicists, economists, historians, marketing specialists) will do it for us. If we don't theorize about our own practice, we're condemned to "be practiced" or to "be theorized." "Without theory," asserts Willinsky, "you risk being practiced by unstated theories" that underlie your day-to-day professional tasks. If it's not your theory, it's the theory someone else, or some other group, will impose on you. It's your choice. It's *our* choice, as professionals.

In an article published in the *American Journal of Public Health* in 2006, Lawrence Green briefly reviewed the history of public health and its sociology and psychology "turns." These turns represented moments in which psychologists and sociologists began showing an interest in public health, in addressing the "complexities of the newly emerging epidemics of chronic diseases" (Green, 2006, p. 406). Yet opening public health to the theoretical thinking of other fields came with important limitations, most of which could only be identified in hindsight.

Among such limitations, according to Green's analysis, we saw public health's willingness to ". . . draw on sociology for ways to measure socioeconomic status, for example, so that we could control for its confounding" (2006, p. 407). At the same time, we witnessed public health's reluctance to ". . . use [sociology's] socio-economic variables to untangle the web of causation that such variables should have forced us to grapple with much sooner."

We borrowed some of the concepts and analytical tools from sociology, in other words, but didn't care to delve into the complex causal webs uncovered by these tools. Stated differently: we improved our measurement and analytical skills, but our theorizing didn't follow suit.

The mark psychology left on public health also came with a hefty price. According to Green (2006),

> For all the enrichment of critical scientific and theoretical thinking on behav-
> ioral issues in public health that psychologists brought, their domination of that
> thinking could be seen in retrospect as regression to the individualistic mean and
> to the reductionist methodologies of experimental psychology rather than the
> community and systems thinking [required by public health]. (p. 407)

Paraphrasing Green's statement, our rendezvous with psychology kept us confined to a worldview dominated by individual-level variables when we needed to be examining public health from the perspective of broader, multilevel influences.

Despite these not-so-perfect exchanges with other fields of knowledge, because public health is an applied field and it is the nature of applied fields to borrow theoretical frameworks from other disciplines, incorporating constructs from various social sciences into public health will remain a common practice. It becomes vital, therefore, for "public health professionals and researchers to *remain critically reflective* about the processes by which social science is trans-lated into the public health mainstream" (Moore, Shiell, Hawe, & Haines, 2005, p. 1330).

As we begin, for instance, to seek help in understanding health and illness from different perspectives such as Social Capital theory, or systems theory/systems science, several theoretical thinkers are proactively asking important questions regarding the scope and quality of the contributions these approaches can provide. Green (2006), for one, asks of systems-type approaches, "Which concepts and methods will be most useful?" and "Who will support this new addition to public health?" (p. 408), whereas Moore et al. (2005) question: "Is social capital a more accurate predictor of variations in health outcomes than economic and income-related factors?" (p. 1331).

Uncritical adoption of constructs, methods, and propositions from other sciences—as exciting and as promising as these new perspectives might be for our own understanding of health—generates not only the potential for hegemony, but also the potential for a dangerous "misfit" between these constructs and the complexities of public health realities. Disenchanted by these potential pitfalls, many scholars are calling, in fact, for "theoretical innovation" in public health (Potvin, Gendron, Bilodeau, & Chabot, 2005, p. 591).

Whether we heed the call to develop theories unique to the public health field or continue to borrow theoretical frameworks, questions such as those being asked of systems sciences or social capital theory and reflections about which theoretical influences we might allow to permeate public health can only be addressed through careful and systematic theoretical thinking. Without it, we would be at the mercy of our own ignorance or resistance, at best, and subject to other fields' ideological whims, at worst.

Reason 5: Because Theoretical Thinking Guides and Perfects Practice

In the beginning of this chapter, I offered a definition of practice extending beyond the mere development, implementation, and evaluation of health promotion programs (see note 1). To understand the fifth reason for thinking theoretically, it will be easier, however, if we focus narrowly on the notion of practice as the *set of activities* we engage in to promote health and prevent illness. Within this narrower view, I challenge you to consider the possibility that theory doesn't merely inform our activities or makes practice a bit more efficient; indeed, "theory makes perfect," as educator John Willinsky proposes (1998, p. 245).

Reviews of the public health literature have consistently indicated that health promotion or prevention interventions are more effective in generating desired outcomes if they are based on or informed by theory (Elder, Ayala, & Harris, 1999; Hochbaum, Sorenson, & Lorig, 1992; Jackson, 1997; Whitehead & Russell, 2004). Some of the better or most user-friendly health behavior theories suggest which methods or strategies work best to influence specific health determinants; therefore, programs anchored in available scientific or educational theories do not have to reinvent the proverbial wheel and do not have to guess wildly about which objectives, means, and outcomes the program should devise. Here is how Rimer, Glanz, and Rasband (2001) put it:

> The development and use of an analytical framework, or logic framework, [for planning and implementing interventions] can be very helpful in clarifying and

communicating which processes and outcomes are considered most important. A logic framework requires that we articulate the underlying theory of the intervention, presumed mediating and process factors, and ultimate outcomes. With a logic framework, the chain of evidence then becomes clear, and links that are already well established in the literature can be supported. (p. 242)

When health educators use a planning model, such as PRECEDE–PROCEED or Intervention Mapping, to design and strategize what their program or intervention will look like and how it will operate, this, in itself, is a form of theoretical thinking: As these health educators plan and map their practice, they are constructing a theory of action (Argyris, 1974), proposing a series of cause-and-effect logical associations: "If we teach cooking lessons to parents, they will learn how to prepare healthier, more nutritious meals for their children; their children will avoid eating junk food, thus preventing premature obesity."

Even when health promotion programs are not explicitly theory-based, that is, they don't invoke a health behavior theory (e.g., Social Cognitive Theory or social support theories) as their basis, they remain theory-based, implicitly. Every intervention operates on assumptions of what works and what doesn't, or which activities (or causes) will lead to specific outcomes (or effects). Every program, therefore, has an implicit theory of action (Patton, 1997).

If theories remain implicit, however, it becomes more difficult to perceive their benefits. Making theories of action explicit, therefore, may save practitioners precious time when deciding which activities they should implement, where to start developing their intervention, and how to make it more efficient. Established theories (because it's taken several years to test them) provide suggestions of methods and strategies that tend to work best for specific populations and in specific circumstances. Hochbaum et al. (1992) described this eloquently saying:

[Theories] furnish us with valuable tools for solving a wide variety of problems in our work. In the context of our professional practice, our theories can be regarded as being essentially statements identifying factors that are likely to produce particular results under specified conditions. To put it in other words, good and proven theories, if well chosen and skillfully adapted, can help us predict what consequences various interventions are likely to have even in situations we have never before encountered. Certain social and behavioral science theories and theories from a number of other fields represent our best understanding of human health-relevant behavior and of other factors of concern to the profession. They can, therefore, be invaluable at times as guides for selecting or developing and applying the most promising strategies and methods in any given situation." (p. 296)

Public health practitioners are shortchanging themselves when they avoid using theory to help develop their programs: Most of the theories used in health promotion have very specific suggestions for how to enhance clients' motivation, how to build people's confidence, and how to help them manage their fears and concerns. Here is an example: When discussing how people regulate their own behaviors, Bandura's presentation of the issue automatically suggests possible strategies for intervention. (In case you're not familiar with Albert Bandura, he is one of the main proponents of Social Cognitive Theory, responsible for giving us the concepts of self-efficacy and observational learning.) Here's what Bandura (1986) says when describing the theoretical aspects of self-regulation:

> People get themselves to do things they would otherwise put off or avoid altogether by making tangible incentives dependent upon performance attainments. By making free time, relaxing breaks, recreational activities, and other types of tangible self-reward contingent upon a certain amount of progress in an activity, they mobilize the effort necessary to get things done. (p. 351)

If a practitioner is thinking about setting up a health education intervention aimed at increasing sedentary people's daily levels of physical activity, by reading this portion of Bandura's work, this practitioner might be prompted to think about how to build self-rewards into his or her program. Perhaps the health educator could lead the program participants to choose self-rewards that they value and could teach them how to manage these tangible incentives to reinforce new physical activity behaviors. For example, one participant may choose to reward herself with a new pair of expensive walking shoes, if she logs in 30 minutes of walking every day for 25 days of a month.

Yet, if practitioners were to continue reading and searching for intervention strategies in Bandura's work, they would also learn that there are important nuances in helping people regulate their own behavior through the use of incentives. One such nuance regards whether individuals *can*, in fact, engage in that specific behavior (e.g., walk for 30 minutes a day for 6 days a week when previously they walked very little). If people are not confident or don't have a certain level of self-efficacy to perform the behavior, it doesn't matter that they have put in place pleasurable self-rewards; the behavior will not occur, and the reinforcement will not be applied. Through familiarizing him/herself with the theory as a whole, its multiple factors, and their relationships, the health educator can then make more appropriate decisions about which factors to target, how best to change these factors, and therefore develop a more effective program.

Having thus far defended the use of theories in health promotion practice, I find it necessary, nevertheless, to counterbalance this defense with the caveat mentioned by Hochbaum in his 1992 article *Theory in Health Education Practice*.

While theories are useful for suggesting interventions, strategies, and which variables to target in these interventions, affirms Hochbaum et al. (1992), theories do not tell practitioners what to do:

> That is why we use terms like, "suggested by such and such theory" or "theory-informed" rather than "theory-determined" or "theory-driven" when we speak of health education programs . . . our theories are merely instruments to help us find (not tell us) the most promising designs, strategies, methods, and techniques in the process of planning our programs, and powerful instruments they can be when selected and used properly. But even the best and most proven theories are no substitute for practitioners' training, experience, mastery of skills, knowledge, and inventiveness. Those possessing these qualities will find theories potentially powerful tools; those lacking these qualities will find them useless at best, misleading at worst. We cannot stress this too much because disillusionment with theories is very often due to expecting from them what they simply cannot deliver." (pp. 308–309)

I agree with Hochbaum's view. While theoretical thinking can perfect practice (and here Hochbaum and I mean practice in the sense of the activities we develop to promote health and prevent disease), it does not constitute a recipe book for practitioners. Nevertheless, practitioners gain much, and avoid substantial headaches, if they think theoretically about their professional tasks.

Reason 6: Because Theoretical Thinking Builds Scientific Knowledge

Theoretical thinking represents the ground in which the knowledge-base of health promotion is rooted, grows, and develops, much like a well-tended garden. Granted, public health promotion and particularly health education are applied fields: They focus on solving problems, facilitating healthy decision making, and providing practical solutions to everyday threats to our health (Rasberry & Goodson, 2006). Yet, public health's attempt to gain legitimacy among other disciplines and to align itself with a scientific, biomedical model (Buchanan, 2006b) has pushed the field in the direction of research—not merely evaluations of health promotion interventions but also basic research on the determinants or causes of health behavior.

If examined closely, however, much of the research carried out in public health is descriptive in nature: epidemiologic studies describing the distribution of diseases among certain population groups (Geanuracos et al., 2007; Lantz et al., 2006), evaluations of educational prevention programs or marketing campaigns

(Cameron et al., 2007; Neuhauser et al., 2007), and outcomes research (i.e., research based on observations and hypotheses not linked to a theoretical model, common in the medical field) (Busch & Custer, 2006; Reeve et al., 2007). Fewer studies focus on theoretical questions or reflect on public health history, its practices, and methods of delivery (Rogers, 2007). In summary, much of the research we consume and apply is "descriptive, rather than analytical, interpretive or critical" (Norgaard, Morgall, & Bissell, 2000, p. 77).

A profession's body of knowledge requires both types of research—descriptive and analytical/critical—no doubt. But development of a sound knowledge-base or the construction of meaning in a given discipline happens only within the realm of analytical, interpretive, or critical (in other words, theoretical) thinking.

I understood this distinction between description and analysis/interpretation better when, during my doctoral training, I read a short story written by Bernard K. Forscher (1963), published as a letter to the editor in the journal *Science*. Titled *"Chaos in the Brickyard,"* I transcribe it here, in its entirety, so you can appreciate its uniqueness:

> Once upon a time, among the activities and occupations of man [*sic*] there was an activity called scientific research and the performers of this activity were called scientists. In reality, however, these men [sic] were builders who constructed edifices, called explanations or laws, by assembling bricks, called facts. When the bricks were sound and were assembled properly, the edifice was useful and durable and brought pleasure, and sometimes reward, to the builder. If the bricks were faulty or if they were assembled badly, the edifice would crumble, and this kind of disaster could be very dangerous to innocent users of the edifice as well as to the builder who sometimes was destroyed by the collapse. Because the quality of the bricks was so important to the success of the edifice, and because bricks were so scarce, in those days the builders made their own bricks. The making of bricks was a difficult and expensive undertaking and the wise builder avoided waste by making only bricks of the shape and size necessary for the enterprise at hand. The builder was guided in this manufacture by a blueprint, called a theory or hypothesis.
>
> It came to pass that builders realized that they were sorely hampered in their efforts by delays in obtaining bricks. Thus there arose a new skilled trade known as brickmaking, called junior scientist to give the artisan proper pride in his work. This arrangement was very efficient and the construction of edifices proceeded with great vigor. Sometimes brickmakers became inspired and progressed to the status of builders. In spite of the separation of duties, bricks still were made with care and usually were produced only on order. Now and then an enterprising brickmaker was able to foresee a demand and would prepare a stock of bricks ahead of time, but, in general, brickmaking was done on a custom basis because it still was a difficult and expensive process.

And then it came to pass that a misunderstanding spread among the brick-makers (there are some who say that this misunderstanding developed as a result of careless training of a new generation of brickmakers). The brickmakers became obsessed with the making of bricks. When reminded that the ultimate goal was edifices, not bricks, they replied that, if enough bricks were available, the build-ers would be able to select what was necessary and still continue to construct edifices. The flaws in this argument were not readily apparent and so, with the help of the citizens who were waiting to use the edifices yet to be built, amazing things happened. The expense of brickmaking became a minor factor because large sums of money were made available; the time and effort involved in brick-making was reduced by ingenious automatic machinery; the ranks of the brick-makers were swelled by augmented training programs and intensive recruitment. It even was suggested that the production of a suitable number of bricks was equivalent to building an edifice and therefore should entitle the industrious brickmaker to assume the title of builder and, with the title, the authority.

And so it happened that the land became flooded with bricks. It became necessary to organize more and more storage places, called journals, and more and more elaborate systems of bookkeeping to record the inventory. In all of this the brickmakers retained their pride and skill and the bricks were of the very best quality. But production was ahead of demand and bricks no longer were made to order. The size and shape was not dictated by changing trends in fashion. In order to compete successfully with other brickmakers, production emphasized those types of brick that were easy to make and only rarely did an adventuresome brickmaker attempt a difficult or unusual design. The influence of tradition in production methods and in types of product became a dominating factor.

Unfortunately, the builders were almost destroyed. It became difficult to find the proper bricks for a task because one had to hunt among so many. It became difficult to find a suitable plot for construction of an edifice because the ground was covered with loose bricks. It became difficult to complete a useful edifice because, as soon as the foundations were discernible, they were buried under an avalanche of random bricks. And, saddest of all, sometimes no effort was made even to maintain the distinction between a pile of bricks and a true edifice.

Each bit of data we collect so efficiently in public health is a brick. We require theory to mortar the bricks and build a structure of some sort. In the absence of theoretical thinking, all we have left are scattered bricks, lying around in big, disorganized piles, building nothing. Theory is the only way to connect the bricks into meaningful (even beautiful) structures that help us make sense of our reality.

One example of how it takes theoretical thinking to build scientific structures from isolated bricks of data is the development of the field of psychoneuroimmu-nology. The term is a mouthful because it brings together elements from various disciplines: psychology/psychiatry, neurology/neuroscience, and immunology.

Known as PNI for short, it sprung into existence in the mid to late 1980s when scientists proposed a new way of thinking about human physiology. This new way of thinking did not separate the mind from the body and did not privilege the brain as the only official residence for emotions and consciousness (Pert, Ruff, Weber, & Herkenham, 1985).

The new paradigm began mortaring many loose bricks found lying around in various disciplines' brickyards for a long time. It began connecting disjointed facts, such as college students contracting the flu right before final exams week in almost epidemic numbers, healthy widows dying of "broken heart syndrome" soon after losing their spouses, type A personalities being more prone to heart attacks, and others. Only when a new way of thinking theoretically about human physiology came about were scientists able to articulate all this information and understand the logic behind each of these seemingly "bizarre" occurrences. Here is how one of the original proponents of PNI, Candace Pert—a scientist who discovered endorphin receptors and mapped the human endorphin system—describes the "building" of this new way of thinking;

> Even with the development of modern psychology and psychiatry, mind and emotions are still not studied as part of the physical body, but are kept apart from it in a world of their own. In keeping with this spirit, still deeply entrenched in our mainstream medical practices, the 'head' and the 'body' doctors rarely sit down at the same table. . . .
>
> But contrary to the reigning-paradigm belief, the body doesn't exist merely to carry the head around! The body isn't an appendage dangling from the almighty brain that rules over all systems. Instead, the brain itself is one of many nodal, or entry, points into a dynamic network of communication that unites all systems—nervous, endocrine, immune, respiratory, and more. This is called the psychosomatic network, and the linking elements to keep it all together are the informational substances—peptides, hormones, and neurotransmitters—known as the molecules of emotion.
>
> In 1985, Michael [R. Ruff] and I proposed the existence of a psychosomatic network that is mediated by the emotions, and we published our theory in *The Journal of Immunology*. It was that scientific paper—along with our earlier research on the connection of brain, endocrine and immune systems—that helped launch a new field known as psychoneuroimmunology (PNI). (Pert & Marriott, 2006, pp. 33, 35)

An entire interdisciplinary field was "built," thanks to the ability of scientists to think theoretically about what they saw in their laboratories in novel ways. Were it not for PNI, our understanding of the role that emotions play in promoting or damaging health would still be relegated to the realm of anecdotal evidence, to the realm of the "interesting" or the "outlandish," and dismissed as having little or no value for prevention efforts (Pert et al., 1985). Thanks to this new building in the brickyard (new kid on the block?), health promotion has begun (albeit slowly) to incorporate emotions, moods, and mental states into prevention programming and research, quite effectively.

Just one example of the contributions PNI can make to public health, among many, is expressed in a 2003 editorial in the *American Journal of Public Health*, authored by David J. Malebranche. Discussing the next steps public health should take to address the HIV epidemic among black men in the United States, Malebranche (2003) proposes that looking into PNI for understanding the issues shaping this epidemic among black males, can be very useful:

> Psychoneuroimmunology—the study of interactions between psychological fac-
> tors and immune system function—has already identified associations between
> mental states and disease progression. For example, for HIV-seropositive gay
> men, traumatic events, such as the death of a partner, or attributions of negative
> experiences to self can predict faster CD4 decline and progression of disease.
> Exploring the relationship between stress, mental health, and immune markers
> of susceptibility to HIV is a plausible approach to understanding the current
> disparity in HIV rates between BMSM [Black men who have sex with men] and
> other MSM [men who have sex with men]. (p. 864)

As with the development of PNI, other attempts to mortar loose bricks in the public health brickyard are currently underway, such as the application of social capital perspectives and systems science to the understanding of health determinants. Continued development of these perspectives will require theoretical thinking of the highest quality. The bottom-line, take-home message is this: For research to actually contribute to knowledge development in public health, theoretical thinking is imperative. Without it, we're left with piles of descriptive bits of data, mere bricks scattered in the brickyard, building nothing but clutter.

Reason 7: Because Theoretical Thinking Provides Roadmaps for Research

Scholars in applied disciplines have consistently asked for more theory-based research because theory-driven inquiry leads to analytical-type studies, capable of going beyond mere descriptions of the here and now, and capable of generalizing results. Norgaard et al. (2000), for instance, when advocating for more theory-based research in their field of pharmacy practice, conclude "we argue for theory-based PPR [pharmacy practice research] because we see a tendency in this field to focus on descriptive studies that address the 'what' or 'how many' questions, but rarely answer the 'why' questions" (p. 77).

Similarly, a colleague of mine who serves as the editor of *Rehabilitation Psychology* had this to say about his expectations (in Elliott, 2006) of articles to be published in that journal:

> As a psychological journal, *Rehabilitation Psychology* places a high premium on theoretical explanations and prediction; in this process, we expect authors will provide studies that advance psychological theory, regardless of the diagnostic conditions that may be under investigation. Studies reporting theory-driven, prospective prediction of meaningful outcomes are particularly encouraged. (p. 1)

Granted, this editor's field is similar to health promotion in its emphasis on practical applications to improve quality of life; therefore, the call for theory-based research is symmetrically balanced with the need to publish studies "that focus on improving quality of life for persons living with chronic disease and disability" (Elliott, 2006, p. 1).

Gioiella (1996) emphasizes that in her field—nursing—theory-based research is a must due to its ability to identify generalizable practices and outcomes. For her,

> Clinical guidelines for much of nursing practice are being and will continue to be developed. These guidelines, to be credible, must be based on sound science. It is, therefore, more important than ever for nurse researchers to do good science, that is, science guided by theory. (p. 47)

Yet, theory-based research not only affects the quality of the final product (i.e., knowledge in the field)—it also makes the processes of conducting and implementing a research project much easier and logical. Imagine a researcher wishes to study the use of condoms among HIV serodiscordant couples (one partner is HIV positive and the other, HIV negative). The researcher could brainstorm an entire list of variables to observe and measure, such as partners' age, education, income levels, knowledge of condom use, knowledge of HIV transmission, duration of the relationship, and so forth, without giving much thought to *why* or *how* these bits of information might help understand couples' use (or nonuse) of condoms in their sexual relationships. However, if the same researcher starts with one or more health behavior theories in mind, he or she will know precisely what to look for and which variables to measure. If, for instance, the investigator chooses to use the Precaution Adoption Process Model—developed specifically to explain "why and how people make deliberate changes in their habitual patterns" (Weinstein & Sandman, 2002, p. 124)—he or she will be interested in assessing in which stage of decision (to take precautionary action) each member of the couple finds himself or herself. If in addition to the Precaution Adoption Process Model the researcher also thinks from the perspective of the Health Belief Model, he or she will make sure certain variables such as "perceived susceptibility" or "cues to action" will be measured as well (Champion & Skinner, 2008; Hochbaum et al., 1992).

Moreover, theories not only provide a blueprint of *which variables to measure*, they also come to the rescue when it is time to *analyze what was measured*. While it is true that "contemporary research emphasizes statistical technique to the virtual exclusion of logical discourse [or theory]" (Aneshensel, 2002, p. 01), in essence all statistical data analyses are designed to test theoretical predictions, or hypotheses. Although statistical calculations may reveal numerical associations among several variables in a particular study, it is only based on what theory proposes that the researcher can determine whether these numerical associations constitute, in fact, "true" relationships in the population being studied. For instance—using the example of serodiscordant couples mentioned previously—the researcher may find that the variable "perceived susceptibility" is strongly correlated with the couple's use of condoms during sex. Nevertheless, the Health Belief Model (from which he or she derived the "perceived susceptibility" variable) proposes that factors such as age and gender may moderate this relationship between the two variables. In other words, the strength of the association between "perceived susceptibility" and "condom use" may vary, depending on whether the partner is younger/older or male/female. Statistically testing for this moderating effect makes little sense if there is no logical framework proposing the effect, in the first place. Yet a data analyst working without a theory to frame the analysis may completely overlook this important moderating effect because his or her data analysis may not have captured it spontaneously (Aneshensel, 2002).

Quite often we think of theories as existing "out there," buried in a textbook somewhere, and we view them as a series of abstract propositions and statements about a phenomenon. If we're preparing a research project, we usually approach theory as something we must fit in our proposal—usually because our academic department or funding agency requires it—and as something only remotely related to the data we want to collect and the statistical analyses we want to perform.

In contrast, if we learned to think of theories not as abstract statements, unrelated to empirical evidence, but as once-upon-a-time mirrors of reality, or statements resulting directly from theorists' observations of certain phenomena or, in other words, if we could understand theories as having originated themselves from observations of very concrete events, we might begin to see how theories might actually help us understand our data, right here, right now. Think of it this way: When you were a budding adolescent, full of questions regarding puberty, dating, marriage, and love, you may have approached one of your parents (if you were fortunate to have a good relationship with them) with questions such as: "How do you know when you're falling in love with someone?" or "Why do I get so nervous when I see Janie, and I can hardly say 'hello' without embarrassing myself in front of everyone?" What was your attempt by asking these questions? Most likely you had many motives, but among them was probably this one: You were trying to see whether another (more experienced) person's "theory" could be useful to help you understand your own experience at that point in time. Your mother may have answered these questions in quite "abstract" ways; you may have felt like she was "preaching" to you about the dangers of getting emotionally involved with someone older or about accepting this stage of your life as "normal" and beautiful (as if there was anything beautiful about embarrassing yourself silly because you can't even say hello to someone without turning beet-red! Oh, well . . .).

You get the mental picture I'm trying to paint here: In applying theory to our research, we are invoking experienced scholars' lifetime of trials and errors to see whether they can help us understand our own research questions/objects more clearly and to see whether we can approach our project without having to start from scratch. We often forget that theories' now-abstract statements and propositions emerged once from direct observations, measures, tests, and adaptations of their proponents' own questions (which may have been, in fact, quite similar to the questions we now are pursuing in our own research).

If thought about in this manner, existing theories avoid, oftentimes, that we move in circles in our research; they provide roadmaps for "seeing" the landscape of the journey we're about to begin. Existing theories will point to which variables or factors we should consider measuring and observing. They also propose potential relationships among those variables and specify under which conditions these relationships show up and in which circumstances they are not present (Aneshensel, 2002).

We deal with this topic in much more detail in Chapter 8. There, we examine the role of theory within various types of research models or paradigms. Interestingly, theory will behave and look different, depending on what type of research you do. For now, keep in mind that theories can be extremely useful roadmaps for our research journeys. In this sense, thinking theoretically becomes a rather useful and practical compass.

FINAL THOUGHTS

I hope I have been able to convince, persuade, or at the very least, intrigue you regarding the importance and the value of thinking theoretically about health promotion and public health. In conclusion, I just wanted to offer one extra reason for thinking theoretically, which I encountered when reading an article by Roald Hoffman (an American theoretical chemist who won the 1981 Nobel Prize in Chemistry) (Hoffmann, 2003, pp. 9–11). The reason is not as compelling and convincing as the ones I offered previously because it doesn't sound very "academic," but it is meaningful nonetheless. The reason is this: If you ask Hoffman (2003) "why think theoretically?" one of his answers would be simply "Because 'Tis a Gift":

> Every society uses gifts, as altruistic offerings but more importantly as a way of mediating social interactions. In science the gift is both transparent and central. Pure science is as close to a gift economy as we have. . . . Every article in our open literature is a gift to all of us. Every analytical method, every instrument. . . .
>
> The purpose of theory . . . is "to bring order, clarity, and predictability to a small corner of the world." That suffices. A theory is then a special gift, a gift for the mind in a society . . . where thought and understanding are preeminent. A gift from one human being to another, to us all. (p. 11)

Those of us involved in education know how good we feel when one of our students or clients has that "aha!" look on their faces, and tells us, "I never thought of it [whatever you were teaching] that way." We feel as if we've given them an invaluable present: a new place in which to stand, a new perspective, which can effectively lead to positive transformations in their lives. Public health offers many gifts to us all—health promoting policies and legislation, vaccines, community health practices. Many of these gifts are crucial to our survival and wellness. May it also offer the continued gift of theories, of sense making, and of meaning attribution. Without these, the survival and wellness of the public health profession, and of the public itself, are at serious risk. Remember Tuskegee.

SUGGESTIONS FOR PRACTICING THEORETICAL THINKING

1. Raise these questions in one of your theory classes, or promote a seminar/ panel discussion in which the following questions are addressed:
   - Is our professional training preparing us to become health promotion *technicians*, or health promotion *scholars*?

- To what extent are we being trained in the methods and procedures for health promotion and neglecting to learn how to ask the difficult, reflexive questions about our health promotion practice and research?
- Are we currently training public health workers to think theoretically?
- What are we learning about theories and theoretical thinking? Are we learning merely to borrow appropriate explanatory theories from psychology, sociology, and economics to use these in interventions with the public, or are we learning to develop our own theoretical thinking as it applies to our own practice?
- Are we abdicating the right to theorize about health promotion to medical sociologists, ethicists, or anthropologists, claiming that because our field is "applied" we are not responsible for knowledge development, ourselves?
- Who is currently developing the ideology to which the public health workforce holds?

2. What might be other valuable reasons for thinking theoretically about health promotion? Can you and a group of your colleagues identify a few more reasons not outlined in this chapter?

3. When was the last attempt to build a new building in the brickyard of public health or health promotion? When was the last time a new paradigm, or a new set of values and beliefs, sprung up in public health and health promotion? Can you identify at least one of these "turning point" moments in the field? What was the resulting contribution from that paradigm shift? Were there any drawbacks to the shift?

REFERENCES

Alderson, P. (1998). Theories in health care and research: the importance of theories in health care. *British Medical Journal, 317,* 1007–1010.

Aneshensel, C. S. (2002). *Theory-Based Data Analysis for the Social Sciences.* Thousand Oaks, CA: Pine Forge Press.

Argyris, C. (1974). *Theory in Practice: Increasing Professional Effectiveness.* San Francisco: Jossey-Bass.

Bandura, A. (1986). *Social Foundations of Thought and Action: A Social Cognitive Theory.* Englewood Cliffs, NJ: Prentice Hall.

Bartholomew, L. K., Parcel, G. S., Kok, G., & Gottlieb, N. H. (2006). *Planning Health Promotion Programs: An Intervention Mapping Approach.* 2nd ed. San Francisco, CA: Jossey-Bass.

Biswas, R., Umakanth, S., Strumberg, J., Martin, C. M., Hande, M., & Nagra, J. S. (2007). The process of evidence-based medicine and the search for meaning. *Journal of Evaluation in Clinical Practice, 13,* 529–532.

Buchanan, D. R. (1994). Reflections on the relationship between theory and practice. *Health Education Research: Theory & Practice, 9*(3), 273–283.

Buchanan, D. R. (1998). Beyond positivism: humanistic perspectives on theory and research in health education. *Health Education Research: Theory & Practice, 13*(3), 439–450.

Buchanan, D. R. (2000). *An Ethic for Health Promotion: Rethinking the Sources of Human Well-Being.* New York: Oxford University Press.

Buchanan, D. R. (2004). Two models for defining the relationship between theory and practice in nutrition education: is the scientific method meeting our needs? *Journal of Nutrition Education and Behavior, 36,* 146–154.

Buchanan, D. R. (2006a). Further reflections on a new ethic for health promotion. *Health Education & Behavior, 33*(3), 308.

Buchanan, D. R. (2006b). A new ethic for health promotion: reflections on a philosophy of health education for the 21st century. *Health Education & Behavior, 33*(3), 290–304.

Buchanan, D. R. (2008). Personal Communication.

Busch, M., & Custer, B. (2006). Health outcomes research using large donor–recipient databases: a new frontier for assessing transfusion safety and contributing to public health. *Vox Sanguinis, 91,* 282–284.

Cameron, R., Manske, S., Brown, S., Jolin, M. A., Murnaghan, D., & Lovato, C. (2007). Integrating public health policy, practice, evaluation, surveillance, and research: the school health action planning and evaluation system. *American Journal of Public Health, 97,* 648–654.

Champion, V. L., & Skinner, C. S. (2008). The Health Belief Model. In K. Glanz, B. K. Rimer & K. Viswanath (Eds.), *Health Behavior and Health Education: Theory, Research, and Practice* (4th ed., pp. 45–65). San Francisco: Jossey-Bass.

Chehab, L. G., Pfeffer, B., Vargas, I., Chen, S., & Irigoyen, M. (2007). "Energy Up": a novel approach to the weight management of inner-city teens. *Journal of Adolescent Health, 40*(5), 474–476.

Chen, L.-S., & Goodson, P. (2007). Entering the public health genomics era: why must health educators develop genomic competencies? *American Journal of Health Education, 38*(3), 157–165.

DiClemente, R. J., Crosby, R. A., & Kegler, M. C. (Eds.). (2002). *Emerging Theories in Health Promotion Practice and Research: Strategies for Improving Public Health.* San Francisco: Jossey-Bass.

Elder, J. P., Ayala, G. X., & Harris, S. (1999). Theories and intervention approaches to health-behavior change in primary care. *American Journal of Preventive Medicine, 17*(4), 275–284.

Elliott, T. R. (2006). Editorial. *Rehabilitation Psychology, 51*(1), 1–2.

Fee, E., & Brown, T. M. (2000). The past and future of public health practice. *American Journal of Public Health, 90*(5), 690–691.

Flicker, S., Travers, R., Guta, A., McDonald, S., & Meagher, A. (2007). Ethical dilemmas in community-based participatory research: recommend actions for institutional review Boards. *Journal of Urban Health: Bulletin of the New York Academy of Medicine, 84*(4), 478–493.

Forscher, B. K. (1963). Chaos in the Brickyard. *Science, 142,* 339.

Frank, A. W. (1995). *The Wounded Storyteller: Body, Illness, and Ethics.* Chicago: The University of Chicago Press.

Freimuth, V. S., Quinn, S. C., Thomas, S. B., Cole, G., Zook, E., & Duncan, T. (2001). African Americans' views on research and the Tuskegee Syphilis Study. *Social Science and Medicine, 52,* 797–808.

Garrett, L. (2000). *Betrayal of Trust: The Collapse of Global Public Health.* New York: Hyperion.

Geanuracos, C. G., Cunningham, S. D., Weiss, G., Forte, D., Reid, L. M. H., & Ellen, J. M. (2007). Use of geographic information systems for planning HIV prevention interventions for high-risk youths. *American Journal of Public Health, 97,* 1974–1981.

Gilmore, G. D., Olsen, L. K., Taub, A., & Connell, D. (2005). Overview of the National Health Educator Competencies Update Project, 1998–2004. *Health Education & Behavior, 32*(6), 725–737.

Gioiella, E. C. (1996). The importance of theory-guided research and practice in the changing health care scene. *Nursing Science Quarterly, 9*(2), 47.

Gladwell, M. (2000). *The Tipping Point: How Little Things Can Make a Big Difference.* New York: Little, Brown and Company.

Glanz, K., Rimer, B. K., & Viswanath, K. (2008). *Health Behavior and Health Education: Theory, Research, and Practice* (4th ed.). San Francisco: Jossey-Bass.

Green, L. W. (2006). Public health asks of systems science: to advance our evidence-based practice, can you help us get more practice-based evidence? *American Journal of Public Health, 96,* 406–409.

Green, L. W., & Kreuter, M. W. (2005). *Health Program Planning: An Educational and Ecological Approach* (4th ed.). Boston: McGraw-Hill.

Hinyard, L. J., & Kreuter, M. W. (2007). Using narrative communication as a tool for health behavior change: A conceptual, theoretical, and empirical overview. *Health Education & Behavior, 34*(5), 777–792.

Hochbaum, G. M., Sorenson, J. R., & Lorig, K. (1992). Theory in health education practice. *Health Education Quarterly, 19*(3), 295–313.

Hoffmann, R. (2003). Why buy that theory? *American Scientist, 91,* 9–11.

Homer, J. B., & Hirsch, G. B. (2006). System dynamics modeling for public health: background and opportunities. *American Journal of Public Health, 96*(3), 452–458.

Hunter-Gault, C. (1997). *An Apology 65 Years Late.* Available from http://www.pbs.org/newshour/bb/health/may97/tuskegee_5-16.html

Jackson, C. (1997). Behavioral science theory and principles for practice in health education. *Health Education Research: Theory & Practice, 12*(1), 143–150.

Jones, J. H. (1993). *Bad Blood: The Tuskegee Syphilis Experiment* (New and Expanded Edition ed.). New York: The Free Press.

Katz, R. V., Kegeles, S. S., Kressin, N. R., et al. (2006). The Tuskegee Legacy Project: willingness of minorities to participate in biomedical research. *Journal of Health Care for the Poor and Underserved, 17,* 698–715.

Lantz, P. M., Mujahid, M., Schwartz, K., et al. (2006). The Influence of Race, Ethnicity, and Individual Socioeconomic Factors on Breast Cancer Stage at Diagnosis. *American Journal of Public Health, 96,* 2173–2178.

Leischow, S. J., & Milstein, B. (2006). Systems thinking and modeling for public health practice. *American Journal of Public Health, 96*(3), 403–405.

Malebranche, D. J. (2003). Black men who have sex with men and the HIV epidemic: next steps for public health. *American Journal of Public Health, 93*(6), 862–865.

Marmede, S., Schmidt, H. G., & Rikers, R. (2007). Diagnostic errors and reflective practice in medicine. *Journal of Evaluation in Clinical Practice, 13,* 138–145.

McCallum, J. M., Arekere, D. M., Green, B. L., Katz, R. V., & Rivers, B. M. (2006). Awareness and knowledge of the U.S. Public Health Service Syphilis Study at Tuskegee: implications for biomedical research. *Journal of Health Care for the Poor and Underserved, 17,* 716–733.

McLeroy, K. R., Bibeau, D., Steckler, A., & Glanz, K. (1988). An ecological perspective on health promotion programs. *Health Education Quarterly, 15*(4), 351–377.

Merriam-Webster. Merriam-Webster OnLine. Available from http://www.merriam-webster .com/dictionary

Minkler, M. (1989). Health education, health promotion and the open society: an historical perspective. *Health Education Quarterly, 16*(1), 17–30.

Minkler, M. (1999). Personal responsibility for health? A review of the arguments and the evidence at century's end. *Health Education & Behavior, 26*(1), 121–140.

Minkler, M. (2000). Using participatory action research to build healthy communities. *Public Health Reports, 115*, 191–197.

Minkler, M. (2004). Ethical challenges for the "outside" researcher in community-based participatory research. *Health Education & Behavior, 31*(6), 684–697.

Minkler, M., & Wallerstein, N. (Eds.). (2003). *Community Based Participatory Research for Health.* San Francisco: Jossey-Bass.

Minkler, M., Blackwell, A. G., Thompson, M., & Tamir, H. (2003). Community-based participatory research: implications for public health funding. *American Journal of Public Health, 93*, 1210–1213.

Moore, S., Shiell, A., Hawe, P., & Haines, V. A. (2005). The privileging of communitarian ideas: citation practices and the translation of social capital into public health research. *American Journal of Public Health, 95*, 1330–1337.

National Commission for Health Education Credentialing. Available from www.nchec.org

Neuhauser, L., Constantine, W. L., Constantine, N. A., et al. (2007). Promoting prenatal and early childhood health: evaluation of a statewide materials-based intervention for parents. *American Journal of Public Health, 97*, 1813–1819.

Norgaard, L. S., Morgall, J. M., & Bissell, P. (2000). Arguments for theory-based pharmacy practice research. *The International Journal of Pharmacy Practice, 8*, 77–81.

Nyswander, D. B. (1967). The open society: its implications for health educationers. *Health Education Monographs, 22*, 3–15.

Oakes, J. M. (2002). Risks and wrongs in social science research: an evaluator's guide to the IRB. *Evaluation Review, 26*(5), 443–479.

Patton, M. Q. (1997). *Utilization-Focused Evaluation: The New Century Text.* Thousand Oaks, CA: Sage Publications.

Pert, C. B., & Marriott, N. (2006). *Everything You Need to Know to Feel Go(o)d.* Carlsbad, CA: Hay House, Inc.

Pert, C. B., Ruff, M. R., Weber, R. J., & Herkenham, M. (1985). Neuropeptides and their receptors: a psychosomatic network. *The Journal of Immunology, 135*(2), 820s–826s.

Potvin, L., Gendron, S., Bilodeau, A., & Chabot, P. (2005). Integrating social theory into public health practice. *American Journal of Public health, 95*, 591–595.

Rasberry, C. N., & Goodson, P. (2006). Health Education. In F. W. English (Ed.), *Encyclopedia of Educational Leadership and Administration* (Vol. 2, pp. 452–455). Thousand Oaks, CA: Sage Publications.

Reeve, B. B., Burke, L. B., Chiang, Y.-P., et al. (2007). Enhancing measurement in health outcomes research supported by agencies within the US Department of Health and Human Services. *Quality of Life Research, 16*, 175–186.

Resnicow, K., & Page, S. E. (2008). Embracing chaos and complexity: a quantum change for public health. *American Journal of Public Health, 98*(8), 1382–1389.

Rimer, B. K., Glanz, K., & Rasband, G. (2001). Searching for evidence about health education and health behavior interventions. *Health Education & Behavior, 28*(2), 231–248.

Robertson, A., & Minkler, M. (1994). New health promotion movement: a critical examination. *Health Education Quarterly, 21*(3), 295–312.

Rogers, E. M. (1962). *Diffusion of Innovations* (5th ed.). New York: Free Press.

Rogers, N. (2007). Race and the politics of polio: Warm Springs, Tuskegee, and the March of Dimes. *American Journal of Public Health, 97,* 784–795.

Simons-Morton, D. G., Simons-Morton, B. G., Parcel, G. S., & Bunker, J. F. (1988). Influencing personal and environmental conditions for community health: a multilevel intervention model. *Family and Community Health, 11*(2), 25–35.

Trochim, W. M., Cabrera, D. A., Milstein, B., Gallagher, R. S., & Leischow, S. J. (2006). Practical challenges of systems thinking and modeling in public health. *American Journal of Public Health, 96*(3), 538–546.

Tuskegee University. *History of Tuskegee University*, 2008. Available from http://www.tuskegee.edu/Global/story.asp?S=1070392

Vogt, W. P. (2005). *Dictionary of Statistics & Methodology: A Nontechnical Guide for the Social Sciences* (Vol. 3rd). Thousand Oaks, CA: Sage Publications.

Weinstein, N. D., & Sandman, P. M. (2002). The Precaution Adoption Process Model. In K. Glanz, B. K. Rimer & F. M. Lews (Eds.), *Health Behavior and Health Education: Theory, Research, and Practice* (pp. 121–143). San Francisco: Jossey-Bass.

Whitehead, D., & Russell, G. (2004). How effective are health education programmes—resistance, reactance, rationality and risk? Recommendations for effective practice. *International Journal of Nursing Studies, 41,* 163–172.

Willinsky, J. (1998). Teaching literature is teaching in theory. *Theory Into Practice, 37*(3), 244–250.

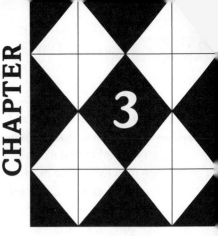

CHAPTER 3

Who Is Thinking Theoretically? Current Use of Theory in Health Promotion Research and Practice

Learning Objectives

When you finish reading this chapter, you will be able to:

1. Name three paradigms for (or ways of) thinking about the relationship between theory and practice in health promotion.

2. Identify some of the obstacles preventing a better integration of theory and practice in health promotion.

3. Tell the story of how practitioners and researchers in health promotion are incorporating theory into research and practice (based on the available literature on this topic).

4. Think theoretically about the relationship between theory and practice in health promotion.

In 2004, while attending a meeting of practitioners involved in prevention programs for adolescents, I happened to comment on the absence of theory in most of these programs' proposals for funding. Having read each of the prospectus they submitted to the local health department, I found only a handful (i.e., less than five) of the nearly three dozen plans contained any reference to adolescent development, health behavior, or health promotion theories. Sitting next to me at that meeting was the author of one of the "unusual" projects that did, in fact, propose a theory-based intervention. In response to my comment, this person remarked, quite matter of factly

> Well, you know, we used theory in the proposal because we knew it would get us funded. Usually, we use theory to "push the buttons" of the funding agency. That's all. But we really don't *use* it to carry out our program. We see no need for theory, aside from the fact it makes the people who give us money, happy.

In Chapters 1 and 2, I proposed that theory and practice are radically connected and even that theory constitutes a *special type* of practice (one that questions both the causes and *status quo* of natural and social phenomena). As you can easily conclude from my conversation with the practitioner, described previously, this is not the most popular view or widespread approach among various disciplines. In many professional fields, the relationship between theory and practice, instead of perceived as dynamic, interactive, and synergistic, is frequently seen as conflicting, problematic, and tense. In this chapter, I briefly outline the three paradigms that have been used to "frame" the relationship between theory and practice (in health promotion and in other fields). I also review the available research regarding use of theory by practitioners and researchers and regarding the theory–practice and practitioners–researchers relationships.[1] By examining professionals' practice related to theory applications, I hope we can reflect on our own theory–practice and identify ways in which we can become more proactive in thinking theoretically about public health.

---

[1] For the purposes of this chapter, I use the words "academics," "academicians," "researchers," and "theoreticians" interchangeably to distinguish them from "practitioners." Nevertheless, it's important to bear in mind that even the distinction between academics and practitioners is sometimes difficult to establish. In certain disciplines (e.g., in sex therapy), many who hold academic positions (such as professorships at major universities) also have their own clinical practice. These professionals would classify themselves—if asked to do so in a survey, for instance—as *both* practitioners and academics.

THREE WAYS TO UNDERSTAND THE RELATIONSHIP BETWEEN THEORY AND PRACTICE

Readers interested in understanding the interplay between theory and practice encounter, in the social sciences literature, at least three paradigms "framing" the relationship and, by extension, the association between theoretical thinkers and practitioners, both in health promotion and elsewhere.[1] Barley, Meyer, and Gash (1988) have done a useful job of organizing and describing these three paradigms, and I borrow from them heavily in this next section (Table 3–1 presents these paradigms, alongside the dialogical perspective we discussed in Chapter 1, in summarized fashion).

The first paradigm is historically the most influential and dominant within the scientific literature. It construes the relationship between theory and practice as one of "diffusion and utilization" of knowledge (King, Hawe, & Wise, 1998). Academia generates knowledge; knowledge is applied into practice. Knowledge "moves" in only one direction: from the academy to the "field." Academics are the authors of this knowledge (valid only if generated through scientific reasoning and methods, keep in mind!); practitioners are its passive consumers, responsible for applying the evidence base that feeds and legitimizes their practice (Buchanan, 2000).

The second paradigm is known as the "political perspective" and is often proposed by political scientists. In this view, the production and dissemination of knowledge are seen as ultimately determined by the political and economic interests that bear upon scientists and practitioners (Barley et al., 1988; Green & Mercer, 2001). For Barley et al. (1988), this perspective maintains

> that scholarly endeavors are ultimately *defined by the interests of those who domi-nate society* and by whose largess academics retain the privilege of pursuing research. . . . The interests of the powerful are said to shape research more sig-nificantly than the curiosity of the researcher, primarily because the former con-trol the latter's access to critical resources. (p. 24; emphasis mine)

Health promotion research and practice are certainly not immune to political forces, and proponents of this paradigm believe that science and practice efforts are limited oftentimes by the types of laws, policies, and norms developed at various levels. Proponents of this worldview would say, for instance, that research on human stem cells and cloning is currently the prime example of how political forces can constrain inquiry and the subsequent interaction between science and various fields of practice,

Table 3–1 Paradigms of the Relationship Between Theory and Practice, Researchers and Practitioners: Characteristics, Barriers, and Proposed Strategies for Bridging the Divide

Paradigms	Relationship Between Theory and Practice	Relationship Between Researchers and Practitioners	Barriers to Integration	Proposed Strategies for Bridging the Divide
Paradigm A: Diffusion Model	· Theory informs practice. · Theory must be "applied" to practice. · Knowledge is generated in the academic/research world (exclusively). · Knowledge flows only in one direction: from the academy to the field.	· Academics generate knowledge. · Practitioners consume knowledge generated by researchers.	· Poor communication between researchers and practitioners. · Practitioners' inability to see the relevance of theory. · Researchers' inability to communicate research findings to non-research audiences. · Lack of incentives for practitioners to apply theory into practice. · Academic training that does not teach how to apply theory into practice. · Lack of systematic marketing of scientific products to practitioner communities.	· Better understand elements of the diffusion process to achieve more widespread and quicker diffusion of knowledge. · Examine and maximize use of communication channels between researchers and practitioners such as professional conferences and journal publications. · Re-examine the quality of professional training, regarding the teaching of theory and its application into practice. · Role model successful occurrences of the integration of theory and practice. · Establish linking agents (agencies or professional groups) to facilitate communication and integration. · Improve technology transfer methods.

(continues)

Table 3-1 Continued

Paradigms	Relationship Between Theory and Practice	Relationship Between Researchers and Practitioners	Barriers to Integration	Proposed Strategies for Bridging the Divide
Paradigm B: Political Perspective Model	· Knowledge is generated as a response to political forces (funding). · Scholarship is defined by the interests of those who dominate society.	· Lacks interaction. · Academics and practitioners compete for available funding. · Academics and practitioners compete for the opportunity to influence the political processes supporting knowledge development.	· Policies for funding research and intervention efforts. · Policies regulating specific types of research and application. · Policies shaping incentives for researchers, academics, and practitioners (such as the tenure-track or promotion processes).	· Reform funding mechanisms for intervention and research grants. · Increase participation of researchers and practitioners in the political and policy-making processes. · Educate policy-makers regarding research and practice issues.
Paradigm C: Acculturation Model	· Theory and practice relate as different cultures. · Theory and practice may have mutually influential relationship, but subject to (cultural) conflicts.	· Similar to cross-cultural relationships. · Potentially conflicting. · Subject to misunderstandings due to differences in language, beliefs, values, and incentives.	· Different cultural norms, values, beliefs, and language. · "Culture-shock." · Cultural prejudice. · Different needs. · Different reward systems for researchers and practitioners.	· Employ "translation" mechanisms (translational science). · Promote cross-cultural interactions. · Promote stronger reciprocal relationship between prevention science and prevention practice. · Examine strategies to promote such interaction during professional training.

(continues)

Table 3-1 Continued

Paradigms	Relationship Between Theory and Practice	Relationship Between Researchers and Practitioners	Barriers to Integration	Proposed Strategies for Bridging the Divide
Paradigm Proposed in this Book: Dialogical Model	· Dialogical: action and reflection cannot exist independently. · Theory is a type of practice. · Theory and practice cannot be dichotomized. · Synergistic relationship.	· Co-learners. · Co-generators of knowledge. · Collaborators. · Team work.	· Ideology: how the relationship between theory and practice has been traditionally understood. · Prejudice: each group perceives no need for the other. · Professional training that reinforces current ideology. · Political forces that reinforce current ideology.	· Shift the process of theory building in health promotion. · Change health promoters' professional training regarding theory. · Adapt the processes of knowledge building (or research) in health promotion. · Take a hard look at the ends and the means of health promotion as a whole.

such as medicine (McBride, 2005). Yet, funding constraints and political forces have long been felt in health promotion research, also (Glanz, Lewis, & Rimer, 1997):

> Concerns have also been raised about the way in which funding circumscribes the type of health promotion strategies used and the specific health problem focus. Some have astutely suggested that categorical health funding (for example, for drug and alcohol abuse prevention, cancer control, diabetes, and so on) is antithetical to health promotion principles and strategies that encourage communities to define their own needs and problems. (p. 447)

In simple terms, the development of knowledge through funded research is a political endeavor: Researchers must follow the funding streams, and individual curiosity or even community needs are frequently secondary to these funding "forces."

The third worldview approaches the relationship between theory and practice—and especially between academics and practitioners—from an "acculturation" framework: one of potential reciprocal influence of two cultural groups. To understand this view, it is helpful to think of two groups of people with very different cultures: Mexican Americans and Asian Americans, for instance. Each group has its own set of values, its own language, its own cultural rituals and habits. Any interaction between them is viewed as a cross-cultural interaction, and as people from one group begin joining or closely interacting with people from the other group, the exchange of values, language, and culture happens.

When we apply the acculturation framework to understanding the relationship between academics and practitioners, we view the relationship as one between two very distinct cultures: science and practice (Rowitz, 1998). The production and sharing of knowledge obeys specific cultural norms, and the exchanges occurring between groups are characterized by the same features present in any type of cross-cultural exchange (such as difficulties with language, different values, norms, and customs) (Frost & Stablein, 1992). Rowitz (1998), for example, describes the relationship this way:

> Academics have difficulty in understanding practice and how it works and vice versa. These two cultures have been in conflict. Academics argue that practice is skill building and is soft in that it does not have a scientific basis. Public health practice argues that it is concerned with real people in communities, and academics live in ivory towers far removed from the realities of everyday life. The integration of these two cultures is critical. (p. 78)

Figure 3–1 graphically depicts each of these paradigms, which I refer to as the Diffusion Model, the Political Perspective Model, and the Acculturation Model.

Despite apparent differences, these paradigms are, in fact, very similar because they all rely on very problematic assumptions. The first paradigm, for instance, assumes that practitioners do not develop any valid knowledge themselves and that researchers in academic settings always know which types of data the "field" needs for its support. This worldview assumes little or no interaction between researchers and practitioners and especially no iterative relationship between the knowledge that is generated in the field (through practice) and the knowledge that is generated in academic circles (through science). Moreover, only one type of knowledge is diffused in this paradigm: that which is generated through *scientific methods* and reasoning, disregarding completely any other valid forms of knowledge, such as that resulting from phenomenological or naturalistic inquiries (I explain these types of inquiry later, in Chapter 8).

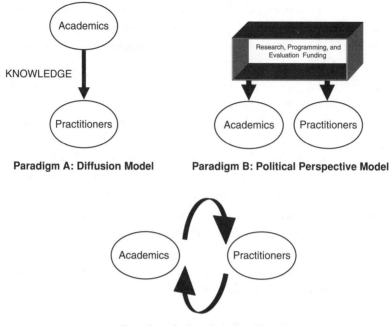

Paradigm A: Diffusion Model

Paradigm B: Political Perspective Model

Paradigm C: Acculturation Model

FIGURE 3–1 Three Main Paradigms for Understanding the Relationship Between Academics and Practitioners (Between Theoretical Knowledge and Practical Applications)

The second paradigm also has its share of tricky presuppositions. The main one relates to how both academic circles and fields of practice are manipulated by political and economic forces into developing specific types of knowledge, and only those types. This paradigm assumes both researchers and practitioners are pawns in political and funding games, generating knowledge through reactive processes only. In this model, there is less room for creativity in the theorizing and researching processes, and interactions between academics and practitioners are, in fact, of secondary importance or even not necessary, as both groups respond (passively) to funding opportunities and agendas that exist "outside" their immediate environments.

The third paradigm, which views the interplay between theoreticians and practitioners from an acculturation perspective, does set forth a more "open" and positive perspective of the interaction. Similar to the other two models, however, it also builds upon premises that, if not problematic in themselves, translate into a worldview fraught with difficulties and potential conflicts. As each cultural group (academics and practitioners) interacts, positive connections can and do occur as knowledge is exchanged, but different sets of beliefs, values, norms, and even differences in language between both groups may represent substantial obstacles to productive interactions.

While only this third paradigm appears to allow for potentially useful theory–practice and researcher–practitioner interactions and takes into account the complexities inherent in the relationship, none of the three views offers a very optimistic model of interaction and exchange. They all frame the relationship as dichotomized and polarized, from the outset, not as a holistic one. The framework I proposed in Chapter 1 has the potential of functioning as a *fourth* alternative, construing the relationship between theory and practice as a *dialogical* one in which theory and practice form a holistic unit, a whole that cannot be safely split apart, or dichotomized, without risking serious loss of knowledge, meaning, and potential for social action (see Chapter 1 for this detailed discussion and for definition of terms).

BARRIERS TO THE INTEGRATION OF THEORY AND PRACTICE

Regardless of which paradigm we choose to understand, the relationship between theory and practice, both academics and practitioners know intuitively there are many individual-level (or people-centered) and systems-level (or organization-centered) barriers to a more productive relationship. Empirical research also has contributed to this intuitive knowledge by uncovering many specific obstacles. For instance, some of the individual-level barriers—or those that reside within the researchers and practitioners themselves—while not limited to the ones below, have been identified by authors such as Buchanan (1994), Glanz and Rudd (1993), Sobell (1996), Morrissey et al. (1997), and Wight and Abraham (2000), as:

- Practitioners' lack of understanding and familiarity with scientific theories.
- Practitioners' failure to see the relevance of theory and research to solving problems.
- Researchers' lack of engagement in the "real world" ("ivory tower" scientists).
- Each group's difficulty in accessing members of the other group.
- Each group's beliefs about the value of their own expertise vis-à-vis the expertise of the other group.
- Beliefs that each group has little to learn from the other.

- Practitioners' perceptions that scientific publications are irrelevant and not helpful.
- Scientists' reluctance to publish scientific findings in nonscholarly venues (such as newsletters, briefs, training manuals, evaluation tools).
- Practitioner and scientists' lack of respect for each other's work.
- The theoretical orientation and training of each group.

Obstacles existing at a systems-level are those generated primarily within organizations as policies or formal and informal rules that govern the tasks of knowledge production and practice. Among these systems-level barriers described in the literature (by Nutbeam, 1996; Lancaster, 1992; Lancaster & Roe, 2000; Morrissey et al., 1997; Sobell, 1996; Wynne, 1996) we find:

- Academic training that does not foster translation of theory into practice.
- Academic training that does not incorporate practice needs into academic research.
- The lack of structured, formal, opportunities for routine interactions among researchers, practitioners, and policy makers.
- The reward systems for both practitioners and researchers that does not prize interactions between the two groups.
- A lack of systematic marketing of scientific products to practitioner communities.
- Research and intervention funding strategies.

In 2001, I conducted my own study of researcher and practitioners' beliefs, self-efficacy, and perceptions of barriers limiting the interaction between science and practice in the field of human sexuality (one of my research areas). I randomly selected a sample of 981 members of the two largest professional organizations dedicated to studying human sexuality in the United States (the Society for the Scientific Study of Sexuality [SSSS] and the American Association of Sex Educators, Counselors, and Therapists [AASECT]) to receive a mailed survey (Goodson & Cheatham, 2002).

Based on specific variables, respondents were classified into three groups: practitioners, researchers, and "both practitioner and researcher." They were asked to rank a set of nine statements regarding potential barriers to the interaction between academics and practitioners. The rankings among the three groups did not differ statistically, indicating each group ordered the barriers in similar ways. Yet it was interesting to note that practitioners ranked "lack of interest" and "lack of time" as (equally) the most important obstacles to communication or interaction. On the other hand, academics ranked as the most important obstacle "resistance to communication." For those who were in the "both" category, the number one barrier was "research findings and theory are not valued by practitioners" (Goodson & Cheatham, 2002).

APPLICATION OF SCIENTIFIC THEORIES TO HEALTH PROMOTION PRACTICE

While less research is available examining systemic elements that function as barriers to the integration of theory and practice, there are numerous investigations of practitioner and academics' individual-level *beliefs* and *practices* in the fields of health promotion, nursing, and psychology (Beutler, Williams, Wakefiled, & Entwistle, 1995; Bostrom & Suter, 1993; Burdine & McLeroy, 1992; Glanz & Rudd, 1993; Lancaster & Roe, 2000; Lorig & Gonzalez, 1992; Morrissey et al., 1997; Neiger et al., 2000; Sims, 1987; Sobell, 1996). Despite these studies' varying foci and research questions, all of them address the relationship between theory/research and practice, between scientists and practitioners. Here is a brief description of what some of these studies have found.

Burdine and McLeroy (1992), for instance, asked nine practicing health educators this question: "How do you use theory in your practice?" A qualitative analysis of the responses uncovered no reports of the use of theory to direct the development of interventions. Health educators in this study said they used theory *indirectly* as a standard or checklist against which they compared the adequacy of interventions. They concluded, "Health education practitioners may not be using theory in the ways suggested by the health education and social science literature" (p. 335).

Glanz and Rudd (1993) surveyed 400 researchers and practitioners in the areas of consumer behavior and nutrition education. Seventy-four percent of the sample responded to a mailed survey designed to assess respondents' views of the importance of central concepts from relevant theories, respondents' familiarity with these theories, and their beliefs whether the theories reflected current thinking in their field. The authors found large differences between researchers and practitioners regarding their familiarity with theories: "For eight of the ten theories [named in the survey], researchers (when compared to practitioners) were more likely to say they were familiar with the theory by margins of 17 to 46%"

(p. 272). The most problematic finding of the study, however, was summarized by the authors as this (Glanz & Rudd, 1993):

> In these findings, a paradox became evident: when asked their general opinions about the value of theory for guiding research and of research for guiding the practice of consumer nutrition education, respondents were usually neutral or pessimistic. This suggests that those surveyed were skeptical about the operationalization of theories for research and practice, and about the conduct of applied research with clear implications for practice. (p. 272)

Neiger et al. (2000) reported answers given by 18 health promotion researchers and practitioners to three questions. These professionals were invited to a consensus conference, sponsored by the Centers for Disease Control and Prevention, to explore opportunities for creating linkages between researchers and practitioners. One of the questions centered on the benefits realized through enhanced interaction between health promotion research and practice. Practitioners viewed collaboration as an opportunity to increase effectiveness of their practice and, therefore, increase ability to obtain funding for programs and to affect policy. Researchers, on the other hand, perceived enhanced interaction as an opportunity to improve research quality and relevance, to facilitate access to communities, and to help build a science base for health education and health promotion.

USE OF IMPLICIT THEORIES OR THEORIES OF ACTION IN HEALTH PROMOTION PRACTICE

If it seems like many practitioners are not using scientific theories to develop interventions and/or to guide their practice in health promotion, it is important we bear in mind that educational or social programs of any kind (including clinical therapy programs) are never completely *a-theoretical*. Even when scientific theories are not employed, practitioners build their programs and practices based on an intrinsic, or internal, *logic*. This logic becomes quickly evident when practitioners answer questions such as, "How does this (selected) program activity lead to this (selected) desired outcome, in your program?" As practitioners explain how the chosen program activity achieves or influences the expected program effects, they detail the logic of cause-and-effect that guided their choice of program activities in the first place.

I experienced a vivid example of this, when I evaluated abstinence-only-until-marriage educational programs in Texas between the years 2000 and 2005

(Goodson et al., 2002, 2004). In this evaluation (which I co-directed with my colleague Buzz Pruitt, at Texas A&M University), we observed exactly what I described previously: little to no use of scientific health behavior or adolescent development theories to develop the sexual abstinence programs. Additionally, as we worked to understand "what was going on" in each of the 32 programs in the evaluation, we found that programs had many different activities. Some programs taught specific curricula to youth during school hours; some programs had after-school activities such as sports clubs, mentoring meetings, community fairs, and summer camps, to name just a few. One program, in particular had, as one of its main activities, the learning and practicing of a short dance routine. The girls who participated in the program formed a "dance group," and they spent after-school hours learning and practicing this routine in order to present the dance at an end-of-year celebration for parents, teachers, and program staff.

The dance activity intrigued my evaluation team so much that we had to ask this program's director what seemed initially a very awkward-sounding question indeed: And how does dancing lead to sexual abstinence among girls in your program? The director, unphased by the irony in the question, did not hesitate at all in answering. According to her, participation in the dance group provided the girls a safe and supportive peer environment in which it was "okay" and even "cool" to be sexually abstinent. As they worked on the dance routine for the end-of-year ceremony, the girls bonded with each other, learned a new skill, remained supervised during after-school hours, develop self-esteem, and were therefore less likely to engage in early sexual activity.

Whether there is scientific support for the director's logic—as a whole—is debatable (see Goodson, Buhi, & Dunsmore, 2006a, for a review of the relationship between self-esteem and sexual behaviors among adolescents), but there is no doubt that the director had a clearly articulated reason for choosing the dance activity for her program. To our surprise, as we asked many other program directors and instructors about their program's logic, the answers were very consistent, and many times, their logic could be supported by empirical, scientific evidence (Goodson, Pruitt, Suther, Wilson, & Buhi, 2006b, describe the implicit theory we encountered among programs).

More often than not, however, "practitioners are seldom aware of their theory of action," says Michael Quinn Patton (1997, p. 221), and evaluators of health promotion programs should be careful to distinguish between what practitioners say or believe to be their logic (or their "espoused theory"—a term coined by Argyris & Schön, 1978) and the logic upon which the programs are actually functioning (or "theories in use," according to Argyris and Schön). When evaluators conduct theory-based evaluations, they must keep these issues in mind. We discuss the role of theory in program evaluation in more detail in Chapter 9.

USE OF SCIENTIFIC THEORIES IN HEALTH PROMOTION RESEARCH

How researchers use theory in health promotion inquiry is also important to observe, but empirical data on this topic are limited. More commonly, we encounter assessments of health promotion scientists' use of theory in systematic reviews of the literature or in meta-analysis-type studies that include an evaluation of studies' methodological and theoretical quality.

In the book *Health Behavior and Health Education: Theory, Research, and Practice*, Karen Glanz et al. (1997) states in the concluding chapter:

> To what degree are professional health promotion and educational activities based on *theory*? Few empirical data on this question are available. . . . In a review of theory use in the recent professional literature, the editors of this book found that slightly less than half of all articles relevant to health behavior and health promotion reported on explicit use of one or more theories. (p. 446)

Other assessments of the health promotion literature have highlighted a less-than-optimal use of theory for guiding health promotion inquiry as well. For example, one of my former doctoral students and I conducted a systematic review of the literature to examine how scholars used the construct "motivation" in health behavior research. We included 44 studies published within a 10-year period (1993–2002) in four health-promotion journals (all with impact factors ≥ 1.0).[2] We found 32 of the studies to be theory-based, but a lack of consensus regarding specific theories led us to identify 21 different theories being cited in those studies! While it is encouraging to find 73% of studies utilizing the construct of "motivation" employed a theoretical framework, it is interesting to observe this lack of convergence or consensus among scholars regarding such a basic health promotion construct.

Another review I conducted with two other doctoral students systematically examined the relationship between self-esteem and adolescents' sexual behaviors,

---

[2] An Impact Factor is a score assigned to scientific journals indexed by the Institute for Scientific Information (ISI). The score results from calculating the times a specific journal has been cited by other journals in the ISI databases (ISI Web of Knowledge and ISI Web of Science) during a two-year span, divided by the number of articles published in that specific journal, during the same two-year period (McBride, 2005).

attitudes, and intentions, as empirically reported in 38 studies, published over 20 years (Goodson et al., 2006a). Only half of the studies in this review had a theoretical framework (53%), and again, these frameworks varied substantially suggesting, yet again, a lack of theoretical convergence.

Trifiletti, Gielen, Sleet, and Hopkins (2005) set out to answer specifically the question regarding theory use in research related to injury prevention. In this study titled "Behavioral and social sciences theories and models: are they used in unintentional injury prevention research?" findings suggest—according to the authors—"few scholarly applications of the most commonly used theories to this important public health problem" (p. 303). They conclude, "This reticence to include theory is particularly distressing given the enormity of the injury problem in the US" (Trifiletti et al., 2005, p. 303). Similarly, Parker, Baldwin, Israel, and Salinas (2004) also examined the application of health promotion theories and models to the study of environmental health and concluded (even though her belief about health promotion interventions is incorrect), "Although many theories and conceptual models are used routinely to guide health promotion and health education interventions, they are rarely applied to environmental health issues" (p. 303).

Several other reviews of the health promotion literature, focusing on different content areas, echo the findings described here and provide some incisive views of the use of theory in health promotion. It is beyond the scope of this text to summarize all of these, but if you are interested, check out these other reviews that either identify the lack of theoretical grounding in a specific area, or call for more sophisticated theoretical thinking related to, for instance, oral health (Watt, 2002), general knowledge-production in public health (Eriksson, 2000), adolescent sexuality and religion (Regnerus, 2003), and health advocacy (Howze & Redman, 1992).

THINKING THEORETICALLY ABOUT PRACTITIONERS' AND RESEARCHERS' USE OF THEORY

Not all studies examining how practitioners and researchers use theory in health promotion are, themselves, informed by theory, but some are. My study of researchers and practitioners in the field of human sexuality was, not surprisingly (given my bias toward theoretical thinking), guided by a theoretical framework. The framework resulted from an analysis of the five most often used theories of behavior change in the field of health promotion, conducted by a team of leading theoreticians and sponsored by the National Institute of Mental Health (Fishbein et al., 2001). These scholars identified eight key variables believed to serve as primary determinants of any given behavior: the *intention* to perform a behavior, *lack of environmental constraints* or barriers to performing the behavior, *skills* to perform the behavior, *positive attitudes* (or beliefs and expectancies) toward the behavior, *normative pressure*, *self-standards* consistent with the behavior, *positive emotions*, and *self-efficacy* (or level of confidence in performing the behavior). Of these eight variables, in my study, I chose to focus on three determinants of this one specific behavior "to incorporate theory/research or practice into one's work": *beliefs* of practitioners and academics regarding each other and regarding theory and practice, *perceived barriers* to the interaction between practitioners and academics, and *self-efficacy* to incorporate theory/research or practice.

I chose these variables based on the following logic: Beliefs and perceptions function as cognitive mediators of adopting or changing a behavior. Through thinking, perceiving, and believing, people anticipate certain consequences (of a behavior or an event) and create mechanisms to regulate their responses according to these anticipations (Bandura, 1986). It is these beliefs and perceptions, or anticipations that determine various courses of action. Beliefs and perceptions are not, however, sufficient to determine a specific behavior. Self-referent mechanisms (or mechanisms of self-regulation) modify the responses to perceptions and beliefs. One such mechanism is people's conceptions of their personal efficacy. According to Social Cognitive Theory (Bandura, 1986), specific skills and knowledge are not enough to guarantee "accomplished performance" (p. 390). Merely knowing about theory and research, or espousing specific beliefs about them, does not ensure that such knowledge will be translated into appropriate action. People's judgment of their capabilities to use theory and research—or their self-efficacy—mediates the relationship between what they know and whether they do or do not incorporate theory/research into their professional tasks.

This logic, however, is not the only theoretical framework applicable to understanding the relationship between theory/research and practice. As we described earlier, Diffusion of Innovations Theory, political science theories, acculturation theory, and dialogical models of the relationship between theory and practice can also offer useful insights into the factors that frame and shape the relationship. Further research is clearly necessary (as much as I despise this worn out *cliché*) to determine whether the factors that have been examined thus far in the literature (such as beliefs, perceived barriers, and self-efficacy) "hold" (exhibit "external validity") across various disciplines, or are unique to selected fields. Additional research is also necessary to test competing theories and to develop a comprehensive explanation of the relationship between theory and practice. Most studies of practitioners and researchers have, thus far, focused narrowly on specific fields of study and have not attempted to develop a general theoretical framework for the beliefs and practices of practitioners and scientists across disciplinary fields.

Finally, another dimension of the relationship between theory and practice that has not been considered *theoretically* is the determination of whether there is, in fact, any *reciprocal influence* of theory, research, and practice in the field of health promotion. In contrast, in the field of organizational studies, Barley et al. (1988) set out to accomplish precisely this task: Adopting an acculturation framework, they analyzed the texts of 192 articles on organizational culture and searched for evidence of conceptual and symbolic influence of practitioners over academics. Their findings indicated that, over time, academics appeared to have incorporated practitioners' point of view on the topic of organizational culture, whereas practitioners appeared not to have been influenced by academicians.

What is the status of the relationship between theory and practice in public health? Who is developing and who is applying theory to public health practice? Who influences whom among public health's researchers, practitioners, and theoretical thinkers? Which group's beliefs have prevailed in the articulation of specific health promotion issues? Careful analyses of practitioners' and researchers' writings—a la Barley et al.—could provide important theoretical and empirical insights into the current status of the relationship between theory and practice in public health. Such analyses would be in themselves one way to think theoretically about health promotion, which could significantly impact the course of our profession. Think about it.

SUGGESTIONS FOR PRACTICING THEORETICAL THINKING

1. Examine a sample of scientific studies published in your area of interest. How are these studies using theory? Do the authors explicitly mention health promotion or other scientific theories? Do they present and explain the theoretical constructs being examined in the study? Do they provide logical explanations of any kind, linking the variables being measured in the study? In summary what is the "status" of theory-use related to your topic of interest?

2. Consider conducting this examination of the scientific literature, following the strategies for a systematic literature review, and submitting your findings for publication in a public health or health promotion professional journal.

3. Conduct a small survey of public health professionals in your geographic region. Using a theoretical framework explaining what leads professionals to adopt specific strategies in their professional tasks, find out what factors may be influencing these professionals' use (or nonuse) of theories in their practice. Include some open-ended questions to elicit whether any of these professionals practice thinking theoretically about health promotion. Ask them how they experience the relationship between theory and practice in their daily work routines.

REFERENCES

Argyris, C., & Schön, D. (1978). *Organizational Learning*. Reading, MA: Addison-Wesley.

Bandura, A. (1986). *Social Foundations of Thought and Action: A Social Cognitive Theory*. Englewood Cliffs, NJ: Prentice Hall.

Barley, S. R., Meyer, G. W., & Gash, D. C. (1988). Cultures of culture: academics, practitioners and the pragmatics of normative control. *Administrative Science Quarterly, 33,* 24–60.

Beutler, L. E., Williams, R. E., Wakefiled, P. J., & Entwistle, S. R. (1995). Bridging scientist and practitioner perspectives in clinical psychology. *American Psychologist, 50,* 984–994.

Bostrom, J., & Suter, W. N. (1993). Research utilization: making the link to practice. *Journal of Nursing Staff Development, 9,* 28–34.

Buchanan, D. R. (1994). Reflections on the relationship between theory and practice. *Health Education Research: Theory & Practice, 9*(3), 273–283.

Buchanan, D. R. (2000). *An Ethic for Health Promotion: Rethinking the Sources of Human Well-Being*. New York: Oxford University Press.

Burdine, J. N., & McLeroy, K. R. (1992). Practitioners' use of theory: examples from a workgroup. *Health Education Quarterly, 19*(3), 331–340.

Eriksson, C. (2000). Learning and knowledge-production for public health: a review of approaches to evidence-based public health. *Scandinavian Journal of Public Health, 28,* 298–308.

Fishbein, M., Triandis, H. C., Kanfer, F. H., Becker, M., Middlestadt, S. E., & Eichler, A. (2001). Factors influencing behavior and behavior change. In A. Baum, T. A. Revenson, & J. E. Singer (Eds.), *Handbook of Health Psychology*. Mahwah, NJ: Lawrence Erlbaum.

Frost, P., & Stablein, R. (Eds.). (1992). *Doing Exemplary Research*. Newbury Park, CA: Sage Publications.

Glanz, K., & Rudd, J. (1993). Views of theory, research, and practice: a survey of nutrition education and consumer behavior professionals. *Journal of Nutrition Education, 25,* 269–273.

Glanz, K., Lewis, F. M., & Rimer, B. K. (Eds.). (1997). *Health Behavior and Health Education: Theory, Research, and Practice* (2nd ed.). San Francisco: Jossey-Bass Publishers.

Goodson, P., & Cheatham, C. (2002). Beliefs, self-efficacy and barriers affecting the integration of theory, research and practice: a survey of human sexuality academics and practitioners. College Station, TX: Texas A&M University, Department of Health & Kinesiology.

Goodson, P., Pruitt, B. E., Wilson, K., et al. (2002). *Abstinence Education Evaluation: Phase 3.* College Station, TX: Department of Health & Kinesiology, Texas A&M University.

Goodson, P., Pruitt, B. E., Buhi, E., Wilson, K. L., Rasberry, C. N., & Gunnels, E. (2004). *Abstinence Education Evaluation Phase 5.* College Station, TX: Texas A&M University.

Goodson, P., Buhi, E. R., & Dunsmore, S. C. (2006a). Self-esteem and adolescent sexual behaviors, attitudes, and intentions: a systematic review. *Journal of Adolescent Health, 38*(3), 310–319.

Goodson, P., Pruitt, B. E., Suther, S., Wilson, K., & Buhi, E. (2006b). Is abstinence education theory based? The underlying logic of abstinence education programs in Texas. *Health Education & Behavior, 33*(2), 252–271.

Green, L. W., & Mercer, S. L. (2001). Can public health researchers and agencies reconcile the push from funding bodies and the pull from communities? *American Journal of Public Health, 91,* 1926–1929.

Howze, E. H., & Redman, L. J. (1992). The uses of theory in health advocacy: policies and programs. *Health Education Quarterly, 19*(3), 369–383.

King, L., Hawe, P., & Wise, M. (1998). Making dissemination a two-way process. *Health Promotion International, 13*(3), 237–244.

Lancaster, B. (1992). Closing the gap between research and practice. *Health Education Quarterly, 19,* 408–411.

Lancaster, B., & Roe, K. (2000). Observations of the past decade's efforts to bridge the gaps between health education and health promotion practice and research. *Health Promotion Practice, 1*(1), 33–37.

Lorig, K., & Gonzalez, V. (1992). The integration of theory with practice: a 12-year case study. *Health Education Quarterly, 19,* 355–368.

McBride, C. M. (2005). Blazing a trail: a public health research agenda in genomics and chronic disease. *Preventing Chronic Disease: Public Health Research, Practice, and Policy, 2*(2), 1–5.

Morrissey, E., Wandersman, A., Seybolt, D., Nationa, M., Crusto, C., & Davino, K. (1997). Toward a framework for bridging the gap between science and practice in prevention: a focus on evaluator and practitioner perspectives. *Evaluation and Program Planning, 20*(3), 367–377.

Neiger, B. L., Barnes, M. D., Lindsay, G. B., Schwartz, R. H., Lancaster, R. B., & Chalkley, C. M. (2000). Unifying research and practice in health education: Analysis and comparison of two consensus conferences. *Health Promotion Practice, 1,* 168–177.

Nutbeam, D. (1996). Achieving "best practice" in health promotion: improving the fit between research and practice. *Health Education Research: Theory & Practice, 11*(3), 317–326.

Parker, E. A., Baldwin, G. T., Israel, B., & Salinas, M. A. (2004). Application of health promotion theories and models for environmental health. *Health Education & Behavior, 31*(4), 491–509.

Patton, M. Q. (1997). *Utilization-Focused Evaluation: The New Century Text.* Thousand Oaks, CA: Sage Publications.

Regnerus, M. D. (2003). Religion and positive adolescent outcomes: a review of research and theory. *Review of Religious Research, 44*(4), 394–413.

Rowitz, L. (1998). Re-engineering public health: the two cultures revisited. *Journal of Public Health Management Practice, 4*(2), 78–80.

Sims, L. S. (1987). Nutrition education research: reaching toward the leading edge. *Journal of the American Dietetic Association, 87*(9 Suppl), 10–18.

Sobell, L. C. (1996). Bridging the gap between scientists and practitioners: the challenge before us. *Behavior Therapy, 27,* 297–320.

Trifiletti, L. B., Gielen, A. C., Sleet, D. A., & Hopkins, K. (2005). Behavioral and social science theories and models: are they used in unintentional injury prevention research? *Health Education Research: Theory & Practice, 20*(3), 298–307.

Watt, R. G. (2002). Emerging theories into the social determinants of health: implications for oral health promotion. *Community Dental & Oral Epidemiology, 30,* 241–247.

Wight, D., & Abraham, C. (2000). From psycho-social theory to sustainable classroom practice: developing a research-based teacher-delivered sex education programme. *Health Education Research: Theory & Practice, 15*(1), 25–38.

Wynne, B. (1996). Misunderstood misunderstandings: social identities and public uptake of science. In A. Irwin & B. Wynne (Eds.), *Misunderstanding Science? The Public Reconstruction of Science and Technology.* Cambridge, MA: Cambridge University Press.

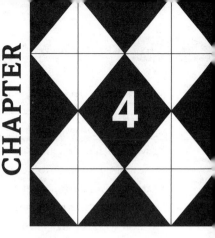

Which Theories? An Overview of the Theoretical Landscape in Health Promotion

Learning Objectives

When you finish reading this chapter, you will be able to:

1. Identify some of the textbooks currently discussing health promotion theories.
2. Name some of the most commonly used theories in health promotion and public health.
3. Distinguish between theoretical concepts, constructs, variables, and hypotheses.
4. Explain the blinding effects of scientific theories.
5. List four patterns characterizing the current theoretical landscape in health promotion.

WHICH THEORIES?

Based on the title above, I am almost certain you turned to this chapter expecting a list of behavioral and social sciences theories you might use to address your research question or to help plan your health promotion program. As if anticipating a wonderful meal at a buffet-style restaurant, you came hoping you might encounter many potentially useful and "user-friendly" theories lined up in neat rows, clearly outlined and explained, ready to be picked, savored, and applied.

Well, I hate to disappoint you—especially this early in the book! At least five other currently available textbooks do exactly that: provide a listing of the most commonly used (and the most promising) theories in health education and health promotion. No sense in repeating the good work already done. It may help to know, nonetheless, that in the latter chapters in *this* book, I will be guiding you through the processes of choosing appropriate theories for your research and program planning purposes and/or developing your own theoretical frameworks.

Then, *what?*—you may be asking. What else is there to cover in a chapter titled "Which Theories?" if it does not discuss specific ones?

To answer your question, I would say there remains the *theoretical thinking type of work* of assessing the frameworks currently used in our field—a rather infrequently attempted task, I might add. In this and the next four chapters, therefore, I invite you to join me in a critical examination of the theoretical world which public health and health promotion currently inhabit.

This critical overview leads to a two-pronged answer to the question "Which Theories?" The first portion of the answer will take us through a panoramic, big-picture view of the theories currently "in vogue" in health promotion. As we examine which theories are popular, we focus our attention on health promotion's "theoretical landscape," searching for evidence of the way public health thinks about health, illness, prevention, and healing. The second portion of the answer to the "Which Theories?" question will lead us to critically assess the weak spots in this theoretical landscape, the areas in which our theoretical thinking remains deficient. Chapters 5 through 8 address these issues.

This is, then, the direction these next few chapters take: first, a bird's-eye view of the theoretical landscape in health promotion, then a focus on some of the theoretical gaps we currently experience, and finally, a challenge—to you—to develop your own theoretical thinking in these areas and eventually improve the field!

MOST COMMONLY USED THEORIES OF HEALTH BEHAVIOR AND HEALTH PROMOTION

As I mentioned previously, at least five textbooks outlining health behavior and health promotion theories are currently available (DiClemente, Crosby, & Kegler, 2002; Edberg, 2007; Glanz, Rimer, & Viswanath, 2008; Hayden, 2009; Sharma & Romas, 2008). Taken together, these books paint a quite interesting picture of human behavior, health, illness, prevention, and healing. We examine that picture closely, in the next chapters. First, let me acquaint you with each of these textbooks, for they represent resourceful tools for your work.

Let's begin with the text that dominated the field for many years (essentially because it was the only one of its kind, for quite some time), *Health Behavior and Health Education: Theory, Research, and Practice*, edited by Karen Glanz, Barbara K. Rimer, and Frances Marcus Lewis. At the time I write this chapter, the book is in its 4th edition (and K. Viswanath has now replaced Frances Marcus Lewis as one of the authors/editors). The first edition was published in 1990. I read it while I was a doctoral student in health education, and I vividly remember a 3-hour, hand-written essay exam covering most of that book's content. The second edition became a required text in the graduate-level theory courses I taught, whereas the third and now the fourth editions remain required reading in my classes. Given how quickly textbooks become outdated and out of print in today's fast-paced publishing world, it is rather impressive to see this text's "survival" for nearly 2 decades. The "Glanz book"—as my students and colleagues are fond of calling it—filled an important void at the time it was published. There was no other text readily available that systematically compiled the most commonly used theories being applied in health behavior research and behavior change efforts.

By the time the 3rd edition of the Glanz book appeared (in 2002), a new text—from the same publishing company (Jossey-Bass)—became available. Edited by Ralph J. DiClemente, Richard A. Crosby, and Michelle C. Kegler, the book was titled *Emerging Theories in Health Promotion Practice and Research: Strategies for Improving Public Health* (DiClemente et al., 2002). While the Glanz book focused on presenting the most commonly used theories in the field (updated, when necessary, with each new edition), the emerging theories book focused on presenting theories and models holding promise for health promotion but not yet extensively tested. The book's authors attempted to broaden public health's theoretical perspective by shifting the focus from what is currently in use to what has potential for future application and development. As of the writing of this chapter, the emerging theories text was still in its first edition.

Between the publication of these two massive textbooks (one has 517 pages of text, the other, 395 pages, not counting indices or reference lists), Barbara Rimer and Karen Glanz authored a booklet, published by the National Cancer Institute in 1997 and reprinted in 2005 (Rimer & Glanz, 1997/2005). The booklet was named *Theory at a Glance: A Guide for Health Promotion Practice*. It summarized—using just a couple of pages per theory—many of the theoretical frameworks presented in the original, larger book. The purpose of the booklet was to have something available for practitioners, a tool that could easily be pulled off a bookshelf and searched for potentially suitable theories to guide program development and interventions.

Despite the availability of these two scholarly books and the booklet for practitioners, many university professors kept asking for a book that could meet the needs of students in undergraduate programs in health education. For undergraduate courses (and for some entry-level master's courses in health education and in public health, too), the texts were not appropriate. So, in 2007 and 2008, Jones and Bartlett (publishers) began to attend to this need and released three new textbooks suited for undergraduate (and early graduate) programs. Mark Edberg authored the book released in 2007 titled *Social and Behavioral Theory in Public Health*. Manoj Sharma and John A. Romas wrote the text released in 2008: *Theoretical Foundations of Health Education and Health Promotion*, and Joanna Hayden wrote the book *Introduction to Health Behavior Theory*.

All of these books fulfill a similar mission: to bring to students of health education, health promotion, and any health-behavior-related field, compilations of theories that can inform their current research and/or program development and evaluation. Personally, I view the books as miniencyclopedias or small dictionaries of theories, where I can find more in-depth information about how a specific framework was developed, who developed it, its main constructs, main focus, and examples of application to real-life problems and issues. As you can see, these are all extremely useful and helpful tools, and I recommend you consult these texts extensively in your professional career.

Journey Through the Dominant Theories in Health Promotion

If you ever have the opportunity, try doing this: Obtain a copy of each of the books I mentioned previously. Line them up side-by-side on your desk, and just look at them. As you look, be reminded that—much like an archeologist who contemplates precious artifacts dug during back-breaking excavations—you, too, are contemplating precious artifacts associated with an important history: the history of your field; the history of public health and health promotion. Together, the artifacts (the books) in front of you tell an important story about health promotion. Actually, they tell several interesting stories, as you will read later on. These books and the theories they contain are products of their historical moments and of their respective cultures. They represent, therefore, well-defined ways of seeing (and of *not* seeing) the world and explaining it. Let's examine then what stories these theories tell and what worldviews they so elegantly represent.

Travel Gear

Before beginning our journey into the theoretical landscape that lies before us, it is important that—as travelers—we equip ourselves with a few essential tools. As your cheerful tour guide, here, I will often point things out that will require you use some special equipment (just as you would need a good pair of binoculars on a birding trip). If you find yourself well prepared for the trip, your journey becomes richer; you can take in a lot more from the landscape and, in many cases, prevent potential problems. Here are three conceptual tools you need to carry with you as essential travel gear when traversing this landscape for the first time: an understanding of basic terminology, awareness of historical contexts, and awareness of theories' blinding effects.

Basic Terminology

Let's begin with terminology. As you navigate your way through scientific theories, you should understand and easily distinguish among the following notions: concepts, constructs, variables, and hypotheses, for these constitute the building blocks of any theory—their fundamental "pieces."

Believe it or not—I guess, by now, you're prone to believe it, as you've seen this one too may times!—scholars have reached no consensus or widespread agreement on how to define and distinguish between *concepts* and *constructs*, even though they constitute "the major components of a theory" (Glanz et al., 2008, p. 27). In our journey through the current theoretical landscape in health promotion, we will adopt Glanz's distinction between concepts and constructs. Concepts refer to ideas or notions that can oftentimes be understood by lay audiences or groups of people who talk about these concepts without worrying about being "technical" or discussing theory at all. The term *construct*, on the other hand, becomes more specialized terminology, referring to ideas or concepts that have been incorporated into a theory and have been baptized with a technical name. For instance, the term "confidence" (referring to confidence in one's ability to do something), in Glanz's view, is a *concept*. Various theories discuss the term, but even outside these theories, people recognize the notion of "confidence" and can talk intelligently about it without even thinking about theory. On the other hand, the term "self-efficacy" (also referring to an individual's confidence in his or her ability to carry out a specific behavior) has been branded a technical term belonging to Self-Efficacy Theory and to Social Cognitive Theory. Self-efficacy, then, is a *construct* because it originated and was coined for very specific use. Lay people would not use the term "self-efficacy" (the construct) to mean one's "confidence" because, in general, they are not familiar with such technical terminology.

I agree, therefore, with Glanz's proposition: *Concepts* are broader notions (may be found inside or outside the theory world); *constructs* refer specifically to the concepts developed and used *within the theory world*. I would be remiss, however, if I didn't alert you to the fact that you will encounter the exact opposite of this formulation in many social science texts. For your information, other authors have defined *concepts* and *constructs* in precisely the *opposite* manner of that described previously. Here's an example. In the book *How to Build Social Science Theories*, the authors propose using the term *concept* for the more specific, technical applications (Shoemaker, Tankard, & Lasorsa, 2004):

> The terms *construct* and *concept* are sometimes used interchangeably, with one scholar referring to a term as a concept, and another as a construct. Differences in the use of the terms *construct* and *concept* center on assumptions about just how abstract the generalization is, with *constructs being more abstract or general than concepts*. (p. 15, emphasis mine)

Despite such variations in how the terms are defined, the take-home message is this: The terms *concepts* and *constructs* refer to the units, or the "molecules" that make up theory. The terms are often used interchangeably, and precision in distinguishing between the two is not very important. It *is* important, however, that you familiarize yourself with the various ways in which scholars use specific terminology; if you're not prepared for these nuanced differences, you may be surprised (or become confused) when you read certain texts or talk to certain scholars.

Now, for something everyone seems to agree with: the definition of the term "variable." Variables, just like concepts and constructs, also constitute pieces of a theory, its basic elements, and here is how the authors of *How to Build Social Science Theories* define "variables" (Shoemaker et al., 2004): "It is at the point of measuring a concept or construct that the term *variable* is used. . . . A variable is a measurable version of a concept or construct that can take on two or more values" (p. 16).

Researchers experience significant difficulties when attempting to observe certain theoretical constructs, especially in the social sciences. Take the construct "gender," for instance. We all understand its meaning, but can we "see" gender walking around, eating breakfast, brushing its teeth? No, gender, as a theoretical construct is not directly observable. "But wait!" You might want to object. "I can observe, rather accurately (most of the time, at least), whether a person is male or female! I can see their gender!" Well, not exactly. What you see and what provides you with some elements to determine whether a person is male or female is not his or her gender. What you observe are the elements, the characteristics, or the "symptoms," if you will, the manifestations of gender, not gender itself. Gender is a concept, a construct, a figment of your imagination (in a good sense, of course). You cannot point to a man and say, "Here's gender." You can point to a man and say: "Here's a man; an example of one of the dimensions of the construct, *gender*." Carol Aneshensel (2002) summarizes this well:

> A construct cannot be observed directly precisely because it is intangible, which explains its synonyms of *unobserved variable* and *latent variable*. Instead, a construct is inferred from its presumed manifestations, referred to as *observed variables* or *measured variables*. The measured variable is, in effect, a surrogate or proxy for the construct. Scores on the measured variable are seen as being produced by the underlying construct, the assumption that links the theoretical realm to the empirical world. This process of operationalization entails deductive reasoning: The conceptual description of the construct is transformed into a measurement instrument. This tool is then used to make observations, generating a set of measurements, which we call a measured variable. (p. 33)

In other words, when time comes to observe, measure, or assess a specific construct (or, for some, a specific concept), than the term *variable* applies. As the word itself suggests, variables are ideas, notions, or factors (factor is another synonym for "variable") that *vary*: Variables vary (ugh! I know, it sounds awful to say "variables vary," but this is exactly what I'm describing); they alternate between high and low, between very little and quite a lot, range from completely negative to absolutely positive, from large to small, intense to mild. You get the picture. If a construct does not have this versatility, this ability to fluctuate between one point in a scale and another point, then it can't be considered a variable. It can only be classified as a constant. In other words, a construct that is fixed—unchangeable.

Think of this, as an example: Usually, the construct "gender" as it applies to humans can become a variable because the construct can vary, on a scale, between two points at least (male and female). However, the construct "male" is *not a variable* because we haven't figured out a way to measure degrees of maleness, ranging from, let's say, "a lot" to "a little." Granted, hormonal measures might point to higher or lower levels of testosterone in a man's blood, or social science measures can assess the extent to which men conform to specific male stereotypes, but what each of these would be measuring would not be the construct "male" or the concept of "maleness." Rather, it would measure the construct "testosterone levels" or "conformity to masculine sexual scripts." Thus, in simple terms, gender is a construct that we can transform into a variable, and measure—the constructs of "male" or "female," however, are usually not considered *variables*. The categories "male" or "female" are usually understood as dimensions or indicators (the signs and symptoms) of the gender construct. (Note: I realize things are not *that* simple, even regarding gender issues; consider the social, psychological, biomedical, and ethical issues surrounding intersexuality, for instance; see Dreger, 1998, for an interesting discussion).

You may have noticed I have not extensively discussed the very common notions of *dependent* and *independent* variables here. I don't want to spend much time on these notions because they apply only to a very small segment of the theory world. To speak and attempt to identify independent and dependent variables makes sense only when we enter the world of positivistic, *causal* theories: theories attempting to identify whether factor A causes factor B, over time. Most of the theories in the behavioral and social sciences cannot easily determine causality, for it takes longitudinal studies, carried out over long periods of time, to establish causation unequivocally (Elwood, 1988). Most of the theories we deal with in our health promotion research and practice attempt to explain how two or more variables might be *associated* or might influence each other. Yes, some of these influences might be of the causal type, but to determine causality with any degree of certainty takes observation over time. It is easier, economically more feasible, and quicker to examine associations among variables: When one variable changes, the other variables also shift. Therefore, for most of the theories we employ in public health, use of the terms independent and dependent variables becomes inadequate.

For the few times you may, however, need to identify the difference between the two, here is a definition: Theories that propose to determine whether its constructs or variables are related in a *causal* manner will designate the *cause* as the *independent variable* and the *effect*, or outcome, as the *dependent variable*.

During my career teaching health promotion theories, I have had many students ask for a list of dependent and independent variables. They become disappointed when I tell them no such list exists and that the labels *independent* and *dependent* are context specific: In one theory, in one scenario, gender may be an independent variable (e.g., in this hypothesis: women experience more depression than men); in another scenario, gender may become the dependent variable (e.g., in this hypothesis: specific amounts of testosterone, in utero, cause/affect the human fetus to develop as a boy) (Hannema & Hughes, 2007).

Theories are not interested, however, in describing isolated constructs or measuring variables for the sake of measuring. Theories are interested in developing a story around two or more constructs. The story's main plot is where the action lies: how construct A influences, or even wipes out construct B, when construct C comes into the scene (in much the same way a writer might develop a screenplay describing a triangular love affair, believe it or not!). The job of a scientific theory, therefore, is to develop a script based on how its basic elements, constructs, concepts, and variables *might relate* to each other.

Because most of what they wish to observe and explain—especially in the social sciences—is not directly observable or measurable, scientists use their imagination to create explanations for what they observe in the real world. Explanations that might help understand the mechanisms of the phenomena they observe. For instance, social scientists may wish to understand why many graduate students experience depression during the time spent in graduate programs. As they watch, question, or even test several graduate students, they are not able to directly observe either the students' depression (only its symptoms) nor the *causes* or the factors that influence that depression. All scientists can do is *imagine* or *speculate* what might be causing the depression and then check out whether their imaginings were correct (so much for the "objectivity" of science, don't you think?).

These speculations about how things *might work* in the real world, these "guesstimates," if you will, are the scientific hypotheses. Again, Aneshensel (2002) states this clearly:

> In developing theory, we construct a hypothetical explanation for a phenomenon by imagining the underlying processes that could generate what we have observed. Note the term "could." We are not able to directly observe that the phenomenon does indeed result from these processes; instead, we merely speculate that it does. . . . Expectations about what should be observed [therefore] are known as *hypotheses*. (pp. 26, 27)

Hypotheses, then, allow scientists to develop the "plot"—the storyline of a given theory. Yet hypotheses propel scientists to turn away from the story itself—from their own imaginary world—and look for clues, for evidence, in the "real" world. If no empirical evidence exists to support these hypotheses, the theory becomes a story that does not accurately reflect the real world. It becomes a rather useless explanation. Hypotheses, therefore, should be the bridge between the mental/cognitive world in which the theory resides and the empirical, real world of everyday phenomena. As bridges between these two worlds, hypotheses are essential theory elements. They help "connect the theoretical dots with the empirical dots" in specific ways. Without hypotheses, theories would not survive: They would have no way of submitting themselves to a "reality check" and stand the test of time.

The Influence of Historical Contexts

Besides understanding the building blocks of scientific theories—constructs, concepts, variables, and hypotheses—it is important to bear in mind another crucial factor shaping any single theory: its historical context. I use the term "historic" here as shorthand for the various dimensions of a theory's context: historic, geographic, cultural, economic, political, religious, and philosophical/ethical. Which constructs or variables receive attention (either through research or as intervention targets) vary according to the times. Here is an example of how the popularity of certain theoretical constructs (and their respective theories) changes over time. The construct "locus of control" (defined as one's beliefs about what *causes* certain events to happen and one's ability to control these events) (Rotter, 1966) used to be a popular concept in health promotion research in the 1960s, 1970s, and 1980s. In contrast, during the 1980s, the construct "self-efficacy" (defined as one's level of confidence in performing a specific task) (Bandura, 1986, 1997) had just begun to make its way into health promotion research. What we observe over time is that locus of control maintains a rather steady popularity, and self-efficacy becomes the new "star" construct. Look at the change in the number of "hits" I get when I search for these constructs in ISI Web of Science, an electronic database of research articles (Table 4–1). The number of published articles citing "self-efficacy" increases over time at least sixfold, whereas the numbers citing locus of control remain rather constant. Determining why such shifts occurred is beyond the scope of this book, yet the take-home message is this: Due to many contextual forces, theories and the viewpoints they express are always on the move. They are constantly changing, adapting, or being replaced by better fitting explanations. Such is the life of a theory!

Table 4–1 Number of Articles Indexed in ISI Web of Science, Citing the Constructs of "Self-Efficacy" and "Locus of Control" Over Time*

	1980–1990	1990–2000	2000–2008
Self-efficacy	327	4013	8080
Locus of control	1034	1765	1367

* Electronic search performed on August 14, 2008.

Theoretical constructs—and, by extension, the theories embodying these constructs—therefore, are a product of their times, an outcome of their historical context. Which factors catch researcher and practitioners' attention, at any given time, reflects the theoretical trends of that period, along with the cultural, economic, political, and hegemonic context in which these variables are used. In the foreword to the book *Emerging Theories in Health Promotion Practice and Research: Strategies for Improving Public Health* (DiClemente et al., 2002), Lawrence Green outlines the powers that, from his perspective, drive the choice of specific theories across time. For Green, the forces determining which theories are trendy, useful, and used come from the *historic-economic context* within which the theories are embedded. Such context often consists of the following forces working in isolation or, more often than not, interacting synergistically (DiClemente et al., 2002, pp. ix–x):

1. The prevailing demands placed on practitioners by governmental imperatives
2. Economic pressures upon the public health and health care systems
3. Epidemiologic pressures of the time(s)
4. Technological opportunities
5. Public expectations
6. Practitioners' personal and training-related biases (e.g., the discipline in which they received their training)

Green's diagnosis of the social pressures surrounding us as public health professionals highlights the daunting complexity inherent in our historical contexts. This complexity—far from overwhelming us—should help us see that everyone's intellectual contributions, even your own, are steeped within intricate webs of interconnections and relationships that define, shape, and color these contributions. Russell Schutt (2006) provides a thoughtful admonition:

> Society is a product of human action that in turn shapes how people act and think. The "sociology of knowledge" studies this process by which people make

themselves as they construct society. . . . Individuals internalize the social order
through the process of socialization, so that their own beliefs and actions are not
entirely of their own making, but instead reflect the social order of which they
are a part. This means that we should be very careful to consider how our
research approaches and interpretations are shaped by our own social background.
(p. 47)

Learning how these forces shape how we currently develop and use health
promotion theories, therefore, will help you become more critical in your choices,
more careful regarding the messages certain theories might embody, and more
astute regarding the potentials and limitations of individual frameworks. Systematically thinking about context will also help you maintain perspective regarding
your *own* theoretical thinking; it will remind you that you are also a product of
your times and whatever theoretical or other contributions you might make will
be viewed by future analysts from the perspective of *your* historical context.

The Blinding Effects of Theory

Finally, as we prepare to journey into the current health promotion theoretical
landscape, it is helpful to keep suspended, in the very back of our minds—much
as we would keep a spare tire in your cars, just in case—the notion that theories
strongly influence our way of thinking in two ways. First, they guide our thinking
in a *specific direction*; they show the way, much as a road map or a GPS system
would help navigate an unfamiliar territory, telling us to turn right at a specific
street or to proceed for 1.5 miles before turning left. While guiding us through
unfamiliar terrain, however, even the most useful maps *blind us* to (or force us to
ignore) other routes and alternative paths. As you focus on following a given set
of directions, you have no choice but *not* to follow the other possible courses.
"Obviously!"—you will say. "One can't follow two optional directions at the same
time, even if they both lead to the same destination!" I rest my case. Precisely
because you can't follow two distinct paths simultaneously (especially if they take
you in opposite directions), you choose one and become blinded to (or voluntarily ignore) the other.

The same occurs when you choose a specific scientific theory to guide your
research or your intervention planning: As you engage in journeying with the
guidance of one theory, you become blinded to the other potentially useful ones.
In this sense, theories not only enlighten, they also bias one's view. (As a side-note:
I realize that in health promotion we often employ constructs and explanations
from more than one theory to develop our models and test our hypotheses. Nonetheless, I would argue, when this happens scholars usually tend to choose from

theories that are quite similar or complementary and their combination also tends to focus these scholars' vision on a certain direction, again blinding them to alternative explanations.)

Pedhazur and Schmelkin (1991) present some interesting examples in their book *Measurement, Design and Analysis: An Integrated Approach* when they talk about theory as "a way of seeing" and "a way of not seeing" (p. 182). Here's one example:

> Barber and Fox (Barber & Fox, 1958) reported on interviews with two "distinguished" medical scientists who "independently observed the same phenomenon in the course of their research: reversible collapse of rabbits' ears after injection of the enzyme papain. One went on to make a discovery based on this serendipitous or chance occurrence; the other did not" (p. 128). What emerges from the interviews [with each of the scientists] is that the researchers' preconception, *their theoretical orientations and interests*, determined how they perceived the phenomenon. Witness a statement by the researcher for whom this was a "serendipity-lost experience":
>
> > Since I was primarily interested in research questions having to do with the *muscles* of the heart, I was thinking in terms of *muscle*. That blinded me, so that changes in the cartilage didn't occur to me as a possibility. I was looking for *muscles* in the sections, and I never dreamed it was cartilage. (p. 135; all citations in this quote are from Barber & Fox, 1958, emphasis mine)

The sciences and social sciences are replete with examples of similar events when researchers—blinded as they are by their theoretical frameworks—become unable to "see" what is "right in front of them," as they insist in searching only for the phenomena described in the theory.

With this notion in hand, as we consider the theoretical body of knowledge currently in vogue in health promotion, we should ask ourselves: What are we able to "see," and what are we not able to "see" within the current theoretical worldview in health promotion? What do these theories reveal and what do they hide from us in our quest to better understand health and illness, prevention, and healing? What stories does this corpus tell?

Let the Journey Begin

Armed with the appropriate travel gear—an understanding of basic terminology, an awareness of historical contexts, and awareness of theories' blinding effects—it's now time to venture into the theoretical landscape offered by the five textbooks I mentioned earlier. To facilitate our examination of these five texts, in tandem, I list in Table 4–2 the theories discussed in each of the books (note that

I don't include the "Theory-at-a-Glance" booklet because it merely repeats much of the content found in the Glanz book). Take a look at Table 4–2; examine your surroundings closely.

- What strikes you as immediately interesting?
- What are some of the patterns you detect from this listing of theories?

Table 4–2 Behavioral and Social Science Theories Presented/Discussed in Currently Available Health Promotion Theory Textbooks

Glanz, Rimer & Viswanath *Health Behavior and Health Education: Theory, Research, and Practice*, 4th edition (2008)	DiClemente, Crosby & Kegler *Emerging Theories in Health Promotion Practice and Research: Strategies for Improving Public Health* (2002)	Edberg *Social and Behavioral Theory in Public Health* (2007)	Sharma & Romas *Theoretical Foundations of Health Education and Health Promotion* (2008)	Hayden *Introduction to Health Behavior Theory* (2009)
· Health Belief Model	· Precaution Adoption Process Model	· Health Belief Model	· Planning Models PRECEDE–PROCEED	· Self-Efficacy Theory
· Theory of Reasoned Action, Theory of Planned Behavior, and the Integrated Behavioral Model	· Information-Motivation-Behavioral Skills Model	· Theory of Planned Behavior	PATCH Model MATCH Model Intervention Mapping	· Theory of Reasoned Action/Theory of Planned Behavior
· Transtheoretical Model and Stages of Change	· Elaboration Likelihood Model of Persuasion	· Transtheoretical Model	APEXPH Model CHEM Model MHEP Model MHEPRD Model	· Health Belief Model
· Precaution Adoption Process Model	· Authoritative Parenting Model	· Precaution Adoption Process Model	PEN-3 Model CDCynergy	· Attribution Theory
· Social Cognitive Theory	· Natural Helper Models	· Social Cognitive Theory	· Health Belief Model	· Transtheoretical Model
· Social Networks and Social Support	· Community Coalitions	· Social Network Theory	· Transtheoretical Model	· Social Cognitive Theory
· Stress, Coping, and Health Behavior	· Community Capacity	· Diffusion of Innovations Theory	· Theory of Reasoned Action and Theory of Planned Behavior	· Diffusion of Innovation
· Clinician–Patient Communication	· Social Capital Theory	· Social Marketing	· Theories of Stress and Coping	· Emerging Theories Ecological Models Social Capital Theory
		· Communications Theory		
		· Community and Organizational Change		

(continues)

Table 4–2   Continued

Glanz, Rimer & Viswanath *Health Behavior and Health Education: Theory, Research, and Practice*, 4th edition (2008)	DiClemente, Crosby & Kegler *Emerging Theories in Health Promotion Practice and Research: Strategies for Improving Public Health* (2002)	Edberg *Social and Behavioral Theory in Public Health* (2007)	Sharma & Romas *Theoretical Foundations of Health Education and Health Promotion* (2008)	Hayden *Introduction to Health Behavior Theory* (2009)
· **Community Organization and Community Building Models**	· Prevention Marketing	· Political Economy	· **Social Cognitive Theory**	· **Diffusion of Innovations**
· **Diffusion of Innovations**	· Conservation of Resources Theory	· Anthropology and Culture Theory	· **Social Marketing**	· Freire's Model of Adult Education
· **Theories of Organizational Change**	· Theory of Gender and Power	· **Ecological Perspective**	· **Diffusion of Innovations**	
· **Communication Theory: Media Studies Framework**	· Behavioral Ecological Model	· **PRECEDE–PROCEED Planning Model**		
· **PRECEDE–PROCEED Planning Model**		· Evaluation Models		
· **Social Marketing**				
· **Ecological Models**				
· RE-AIM Model (for evaluation of theory-based interventions)				

After a cursory examination, one can't help but quickly notice the *substantial overlap* among the theories. I highlighted the theories appearing in more than one book in bold text; you will notice most of the table's text is in bold font. Such overlap represents the first story these theories tell us, and the story is this: Certain theories dominate the theoretical landscape in health promotion, even though public health practitioners and researchers have a considerable number of options to choose from. Alongside what you see in the five books, a review of health education theories published in 2004 also points to some of the same theories displayed in Table 4–2, as the most commonly used frameworks prior to 2004.

The review identified the Transtheoretical Model/Stages of Change Theory, the Theory of Reasoned Action/Theory of Planned Behavior, and Social Cognitive Theory as the three most commonly used theoretical frameworks identified in five of the top journals in health education in the year 2003 (DeBarr, 2004).

The DiClemente book stands out in Table 4–2 as a text that doesn't overlap with the others quite as much. Understandably, it focuses on theories that are only now beginning to capture the imaginations of scholars in public health. One interesting question to ask then is whether the theories in the DiClemente book will eventually dominate the field in the future and how long it will take them to achieve a dominant status. It will be intriguing to see whether a review of health promotion literature, published, for instance, in the year 2020 (perhaps with you as the main author?) will highlight some of the theories described in the DiClemente book as commonly used frameworks.

So, the substantial overlap and focus on a handful of common theories is something that sort of "jumps out at you" from Table 4–2. Now, how about the *patterns* these theories, if taken together, seem to build? In other words, what do you think these theories have *in common* besides their use in health promotion research and behavior change efforts?

Don't feel frustrated if you do not see many commonalities among the theories. You may not yet be very familiar with them or at least not familiar enough to be able to quickly compare and contrast them. No worries. I will point you to what I believe is important to notice now; you can confirm what I'm proposing here as you learn more about each theory.

Several important patterns emerge from looking at these theories as a "body," and these patterns converge to paint a specific picture of our professional field. This picture tells a story of how our profession views and characterizes human health, behavior change, health behaviors, and prevention of illness. In the next few chapters, I discuss three patterns characterizing this theoretical landscape:

1. An exaggerated focus on individual-level factors
2. An undue emphasis on rationality
3. A deliberate privileging of linearity

As we examine each of these patterns, you will begin to "see" the worldviews these theories reveal and which worldviews these theories blind us to; you will begin to reflect on where the health promotion field is weak in theory and which theories and theoretical worldviews still need to be developed. While I guide you through this theoretical landscape, I bear a chronic hope that *you* will become motivated to think theoretically about health promotion and make a conscious effort to improve the theoretical worldview of health promotion and public health. With this in mind, let our journey begin. . . .

SUGGESTIONS FOR PRACTICING THEORETICAL THINKING

1. Make it a point to familiarize yourself with the textbooks I mentioned in this chapter if you haven't done so already.
2. As you examine the theories that have become popular in health promotion, discuss with your colleagues, and generate a list of potential reasons for their popularity (if you're familiar with the theories). If you're not familiar with each theory, "guesstimate" some of these reasons.
3. Carry out a small survey of your colleagues and faculty: Bring them the list of the most commonly taught theories (copy from Table 4–2 in this chapter if you'd like), and ask them to identify some theories they believe might be missing from this list. Ask them also why they believe these theories are in fact missing.

REFERENCES

Aneshensel, C. S. (2002). *Theory-Based Data Analysis for the Social Sciences*. Thousand Oaks, CA: Pine Forge Press.

Bandura, A. (1986). *Social Foundations of Thought and Action: A Social Cognitive Theory*. Englewood Cliffs, NJ: Prentice Hall.

Bandura, A. (1997). *Self-Efficacy: The Exercise of Control*. New York: W.H. Freeman and Company.

Barber, B., & Fox, R. C. (1958). The case of the floppy-eared rabbits: an instance of serendipity gained and serendipity lost. *American Journal of Sociology, 64,* 128–136.

DeBarr, K. A. (2004). A review of current health education theories. *Californian Journal of Health Promotion, 2*(1), 74–87.

DiClemente, R. J., Crosby, R. A., & Kegler, M. C. (Eds.). (2002). *Emerging Theories in Health Promotion Practice and Research: Strategies for Improving Public Health*. San Francisco: Jossey-Bass.

Dreger, A. D. (1998). "Ambiguous sex": or ambivalent medicine? Ethical issues in the treatment of intersexuality. *The Hastings Center Report, 28*(3), 23–35.

Edberg, M. (2007). *Social and Behavioral Theory in Public Health*. Sudbury, MA: Jones and Bartlett Publishers.

Elwood, J. M. (1988). *Causal Relationships in Medicine: A Practical System for Critical Appraisal* (1992 paperback ed.). Oxford: Oxford University Press.

Glanz, K., Rimer, B. K., & Viswanath, K. (2008). *Health Behavior and Health Education: Theory, Research, and Practice* (4th ed.). San Francisco: Jossey-Bass.

Hannema, S. E., & Hughes, I. A. (2007). Regulation of wolffian duct development. *Hormone Research, 67*(3), 142–151.

Hayden, J. (2009). *Introduction to Health Behavior Theory*. Sudbury, MA: Jones and Bartlett Publishers.

Pedhazur, E. J., & Schmelkin, L. P. (1991). *Measurement, Design and Analysis: An Integrated Approach*. Hillsdale, NJ: Lawrence Erlbaum Associates, Publishers.

Rimer, B. K., & Glanz, K. (1997/2005). *Theory at a Glance: A Guide for Health Promotion Practice* (2nd ed.). Washington, DC: U.S. Department of Health and Human Services; National Institutes of Health; National Cancer Institute.

Rotter, J. B. (1966). Generalized expectancies for internal versus external control of reinforcement. *Psychological Monographs, 80*(1), 1–28.

Schutt, R. K. (2006). *Investigating the Social World: The Process and Practice of Research* (5th ed.). Thousand Oaks, CA: Sage Publications.

Sharma, M., & Romas, J. A. (2008). *Theoretical Foundations of Health Education and Health Promotion*. Sudbury, MA: Jones and Bartlett Publishers.

Shoemaker, P. J., Tankard Jr., J. W., & Lasorsa, D. L. (2004). *How to Build Social Science Theories*. Thousand Oaks, CA: Sage Publications.

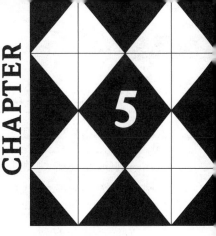

CHAPTER 5

Pattern 1: Exaggerated Focus on Individual-Level Factors: Too Much of a Good Thing?

Learning Objectives

When you finish reading this chapter, you will be able to:

1. Describe the various *levels of theory* used in health promotion.
2. Characterize individual-level theories and the types of constructs these theories emphasize.
3. Discuss what individual-level theories say about health promotion's views of human health, illness, prevention, and treatment.
4. Propose an alternative to the exaggerated focus on individual-level theories we currently experience, in health promotion.

FOCUS ON INDIVIDUALS

After we become familiar with the "dominant" health promotion theories, one of the first patterns we observe is this: Most theories focus on *individuals,* or on person-centered factors. Before we plunge into deciphering this pattern and its meanings, a side note is in order: The term "individual," when used to refer to "persons," constitutes bad English, according to psychologist Paul J. Silvia (2007). He cautions:

> Some individuals, when writing individual papers on various individual topics, refer to *a person* as *an individual* and to *people as individuals.* These people forget that *individual* is vague: Consider "We observed an individual _____." Should the blank be filled with a noun (e.g., rabbit) or with a verb (e.g., walking)? You don't say *individual* and *individuals* when discussing research with your friends, so why be so shoddy when describing it to the vast world of science? Were you attracted to psychology [or health promotion] because you were interested in individuals and enjoyed individuals-watching? Choose good words, like *person* and *people.* (p. 63)

I will take Silvia's admonition to heart and try to the best of my ability to avoid the term "individual-level" as it applies to theories, but this has been commonly used terminology in the field. Perhaps, "intrapersonal" works better in the case of theory and its levels, but I'm not quite sure. I just thought you should be forewarned, in case you worry about the quality of your writing: Avoid the use of the term individual to refer to people or persons whenever possible. Let the public health field know it is weak, not only in theoretical thinking, but in mastering English vernacular, as well. It is surprising, how many weaknesses we hide within our wells of knowledge, isn't it?

Returning to the theories outlined in Table 4–2: Count how many focus on intrapersonal factors (or traits, or a person's characteristics). You'll find that most theories elaborate on a person's *self-efficacy, intention, attitudes,* and *perception of risk,* among others. A smaller number of the theories deal with interpersonal-level variables (e.g., Communication Theories and Social Networks), with organization-level constructs (e.g., Community and Organizational Change), or with political, economical or policy factors (e.g., Social Capital Theory and Political Economy theories).

Levels of Theory

Because I've begun to use the labels *interpersonal, organizational,* and *political,* before we go much further into the chapter, it may be useful to briefly review the *levels of constructs or factors* health promotion theories deal with. I define the term "level" here as different ways of looking at people and the systems within which they are embedded. What distinguishes one level from the other is the degree of complexity inherent in each one (Kok, Gottlieb, Commers, & Smerecnik, 2008, p. 438). Broadly, we categorize health promotion theories as focusing on one of the following levels:

- *Intrapersonal level:* Theories focusing on intrapersonal factors explain health (and illness) as resulting from a person's biological, physiological, and psychological traits. For instance, they explain health and illness as an outcome of one's genes or genotype or as a result of personal behavior and lifestyle choices, motivation levels, and confidence to change unhealthy behaviors. Examples of intrapersonal (or individual-level) theories are the Health Belief Model and the Theory of Planned Behavior.
- *Interpersonal level:* Theories focusing on interpersonal factors provide explanations about health and illness centering on the social interactions between two or more people and how these interactions may influence their well-being. Examples of interactions with potential for influencing health include peer pressure, social support, social networks, and mass media communication. Interpersonal theories include Social Cognitive Theory and Social Influence and Interpersonal Communication theories.
- *Institutional/organizational level:* Theories focusing on institutional or organizational factors focus on elements that characterize organizations and on interactions among organizations that may impact health behaviors of specific populations and individual people (e.g., organizational culture, communication among organizations, and management of health care organizations). Organizational Change theories exemplify this category.
- *Community level:* Theories focusing on community factors explain health and well-being as influenced by the relationships among organizations and institutions in a given social group and how these relationships affect the health of that group's population (e.g., the level of trust between the community members and the institutions that serve them or between people in communities and their schools, churches, banks, hospitals). Examples of this type of theory include Community Organization and Community Building models as well as Community Coalitions and Community Capacity models.
- *Public policy level:* Theories focusing on policy factors center on local, state, national, and international laws and policies with the potential to impact and modify health behaviors of populations and its members (e.g., smoking

and drug policies, alcohol consumption policies, immigration, and trafficking laws). Political economy can be an example (albeit not perfect) of public policy theories.

Table 5–1 categorizes the theories outlined in Chapter 4, according to these various levels.

While this seems to be the most accepted classification of health promotion theories according to the levels on which they focus, different ways to catalogue these levels have been proposed by various authors, as you might well expect. Some (see Kok et al., 2008) propose adding levels such as "society" and "supra-national." Given the globalization of the world's economy and culture, it may now be useful to have the level of global issues of health promotion, as part of any classification (for an example of how globalization issues can significantly impact humans' sexual health, see Padilla, Hirsch, Munoz-Laboy, Sember, & Parkers, 2008).

Table 5–1 Levels of Factors Addressed by Health Promotion Theories

Levels (or Types) of Factors Addressed	Examples of Theories Addressing Various Levels of Factors
Intrapersonal	· Health Belief Model
	· Theory of Reasoned Action
	· Theory of Planned Behavior
	· Integrated Behavioral Model
	· Transtheoretical Model and Stages of Change
	· Precaution Adoption Process Model
	· Information–Motivation–Behavioral Skills Model
	· Self-Efficacy Theory
	· Attribution Theory
Interpersonal	· Social Cognitive Theory
	· Social Networks and Social Support
	· Stress, Coping, and Health Behavior
	· Clinician–Patient Communication
	· Elaboration Likelihood Model of Persuasion
	· Authoritative Parenting Model
	· Natural Helper Models
Institutional/Organizational	· Theories of Organizational Change
	· Conservation of Resources Theory

(continues)

Table 5–1 Continued

Levels (or Types) of Factors Addressed	Examples of Theories Addressing Various Levels of Factors
Community and Groups	· Community Organization and Community Building Models
	· Diffusion of Innovations Theory
	· Communication Theory: Media Studies Framework
	· Social Marketing/Prevention Marketing
	· Community Coalitions
	· Community Capacity
	· Social Capital Theory
	· Anthropology and Culture Theory
	· Freire's Model of Adult Education
Public Policy	· Political Economy

Exaggerated Focus on Intrapersonal Theories

If we return to Tables 4–2 and 5–1 after reviewing these various levels, we notice how theories focusing on *persons* densely "populate" our theoretical landscape: Most theories listed in these tables focus their attention on individual people (in isolation) or on interactions among people (in Table 5–1 you can easily see the majority of the theories listed fall within the intrapersonal and interpersonal categories).

This exaggerated attention paid to intrapersonal factors is not a recent phenomenon by any means. In a classic article published in 1988 titled "An Ecological Perspective on Health Promotion Programs," authors Kenneth R. McLeroy, Daniel Bibeau, Allan Steckler, and Karen Glanz (1988) (yes, the same Karen Glanz of the Glanz book) already raised the issue of excessive focus on *individuals* (my apologies for the bad English). As they reviewed the then-prevalent models and theories employed in health promotion, they concluded many were borrowed from psychology and aimed at changing persons (one at a time, in isolation), not social structures or social norms. Even when the models used in programming efforts contained other levels of influence, such as social support, peer pressure, or even mass media campaigns, the expected outcome was a change in *persons'* attitudes, knowledge, and behavior. According to those authors,

> Even when programs incorporate social influences as part of the intervention—such as peer counseling programs—the purpose is to change individuals, rather than to modify the social environment. Adolescents are trained to resist interpersonal influences related to smoking, rather than attempting to modify the

norms and values that adolescents' cliques, networks or families have about smoking. These interventions may reflect the implicit assumption that the proximal causes of behavior and/or mechanisms for producing behavioral changes lie within the individual, rather than in the social environment. (McLeroy et al., 1988, p. 356)

Understanding intra or interpersonal factors with the potential to influence people's health behaviors is not in itself a problem. What becomes problematic, however, is this *overemphasis* on person-level explanations/theories we have witnessed consistently across most of health promotion's history in the United States. The weight given to intrapersonal theories begs the questions, "What does a theoretical body of knowledge that focuses heavily on individual-level traits and characteristics suggest? What are we seeing and what are we being blinded to by focusing so overtly on person-centered theories?"

The Blind Spots of Intrapersonal Theories

It might be easier to understand the worldview these individual-level theories portray if we start by focusing on what we're *not seeing*. The inordinate value placed on individual-level theories creates three significant (and potentially dangerous) blind spots. First, it assumes an individual person is a separate, distinct, isolated entity. It assumes the concept *individual* actually exists in the real world (even as it remains bad English): It presupposes what we see when we look at people, abstracted from their social groups, institutions, and populations, is a true *individual*, naked, so to speak, with no social or environmental coverings. Such assumption blinds us to a most basic fact: the sheer difficulty in defining what constitutes an individual. How do scholars even define *individual*, apart from all the external forces and influences that shape each person's individuality? Mark Edberg (2007) reminds us of this point in his book *Social and Behavioral Theory in Public Health*:

> What *Is* an Individual?
> Here's a philosophical question for you: Just what is an individual?
> You may think this is a no-brainer. An individual, you say, is like me, an autonomous self that has a distinct physical unity (me, my body, and I), a personality, a way of talking, a way of walking, my own goals, my own motivations, and the ability to plan, initiate, and carry out action. You know, ME.
> Okay, but let's just look at that for a second. We can start with that body of yours. Your physical being, as you know, is genetic—it comes from parents and other ancestors. So, yes, it's you, but, it's kind of them too. Now let's go to that personality. Some of that may have genetic influences too. But your personality, your way of talking, walking, dressing, and all that . . . you didn't think all of

that up from scratch, did you? You got it from somewhere. Just like the musician who is called a "unique" sax player, you pulled together pieces of "how to be," kind of like those riffs on the sax. You put them together in your own way. But most of those pieces didn't magically appear. They came from the social and cultural world around you, including your family; the examples of "how to be male" or "how to be female" that you saw in your personal life; on television, videos, or film; from the tales, stories, songs, and other narratives about people who were good versus people who were not; what a good life consists of; lessons and advice from family, community, and faith organizations; people you have seen who have a style or a "look" that you like and want to emulate; and so on!

It's not so easy to draw a clear line between yourself and everyone else. Of course you take all these influences and shape them, "inhabit" them as your individual life. Yet this process inexorably connects you to your world, and complicates easy descriptions of individual behavior and motivation. Think about this when we discuss the individual behavior theories in this chapter. (p. 36)

The second blind spot generated by this overemphasis on individual-level theories is this: The strong effects (at times, the *stronger* effects) environmental factors can exert on the health of a population are—for all practical purposes—erased from view. When focusing exclusively on personal traits or characteristics, researchers and practitioners easily lose sight that both *natural environments* (such as weather, climate, and geography) and *built environments* (such as houses, parks, roadways, or even socially constructed environments, such as cliques and families) can and do influence health behaviors (Sallis & Owen, 2002).

In an interesting analysis of the application of ecological or multilevel models to health promotion, Sallis and Owen (2002) highlight an important nuance related to who has and who has not been able to "see" beyond individual-level factors. According to these authors, public health professionals responsible for recommending public policies within "national and international health agencies" have been able to avoid being blinded by the exaggerated focus on intrapersonal factors. These agencies, for instance, have focused on promoting changes such as "eliminating tobacco product advertising, increasing the miles of walking or cycling paths available in communities, and increasing the number of low-fat food items available in the mass food supply" (Sallis & Owen, 2002, p. 405).

Yet public health *researchers* have not been very successful at avoiding the blinding effects of individual-level theories. Concerned with this, Sallis and Owen (2002) sound the alert and call for research focusing systematically on environmental factors and their relationship to health behaviors:

Environmental interventions are starting to be implemented widely in the absence of data on their intended and unintended outcomes. . . . In general, we advocate applying ecological models to the design of health promotion programs, but we are concerned that premature or uninformed applications that lead to disappointing results could cause a complete rejection of environmental change approaches before these approaches are adequately tested. Thus, it is important to explicitly identify, develop, and test the ecologically based hypotheses that now play a key role in guiding local health promotion practice and national and international health promotion policies. (p. 406)

Such a paradoxical situation might generate interesting results: a case in which the policy-left-hand doesn't know what the research-right-hand is doing and vice versa. So much for evidence-based practice, right?

Another, but related, serious blind spot is an ethical/political one: Laying the responsibility for healthy decisions, behaviors, and lifestyle changes at the doorstep of the person can easily lead to a "blaming the victim" mentality when the outcomes are less than optimal (McLeroy et al., 1988). When one's health fails, those who believe health is merely the outcome of personal choices and habits will be quick to conclude it is *that person's own fault* for experiencing illness. Therefore, too much emphasis on individual-level factors can, in fact, nurture a victim-blaming mentality (the complete opposite of what health promotion principles try to promote!) (Hancock, 1991; McLeroy et al., 1988).

McLeroy et al. (1988) discuss how an "ideology of individual responsibility" engenders this blinding effect:

> The complexities of social causation are only beginning to be explored [in health promotion]. The ideology of individual responsibility, however, inhibits that understanding and substitutes instead an unrealistic behavioral model. It both ignores what is known about human behavior and minimizes the importance of evidence about the environmental assault on health. It instructs people to be individually responsible at a time when they are becoming less capable as individuals of controlling their total health environment. (p. 352)

Marshall Becker (1986), in his now classic and provoking article "The Tyranny of Health Promotion," also admonishes: "We . . . should stop blaming the victim. It has taken centuries to convince people to relocate the basis of disease in science rather than in sin; health promotion should not be the vehicle that undermines such progress" (p. 21).

The Stories Intrapersonal Theories Tell

Okay. So these individual-focused theories blind us to the potential effects of environments on human health and to the potential dangers of promoting a "blaming the victim" mentality. What is it then that these theories reveal? What do we *see*? What stories *do* these theories tell about human health, illness, prevention, and treatment? You will develop a more thorough answer to this question as you read through the remainder of this chapter and through the next three chapters. For now, it is enough to say these theories are *incomplete*. They prize individuals' behaviors more than any other factor because these theories assume that people have control over their own lives and that each person is responsible for the choices he or she makes. These theories also presuppose human behavior is measurable, predictable, generalizable (or nearly "universal") and, barring minor external influences, manifests itself in very similar ways among all types of people. In other words, these theories tell a story of human behavior (health behavior, in particular) as something that can be studied, analyzed, and understood from a scientific perspective using scientific methods (i.e., observation and measurement). These theories also presuppose and affirm that only those aspects of behavior that can, indeed, be studied through scientific methods have any value for health promotion and disease prevention. As we well know from our own personal experiences and from professional trials, human behavior doesn't lend itself so easily to such minimizing attempts (Buchanan, 2000).

AN ALTERNATIVE—ECOLOGICAL MODELS AND SYSTEMS SCIENCE APPROACHES TO HEALTH PROMOTION

This undue emphasis on individual-level determinants and its concomitant "blind spots" have been highlighted, discussed, and critiqued by several public health scholars. Most appropriately, Buchanan (2000) reminds us that

> A dissident stream of researchers and practitioners has periodically challenged the idea that the mission of health education is to change individual behavior, but these views have had little impact on federal research priorities, government planning documents, or the allocation of program dollars. (p. 3)

Among this "dissident stream of researchers and practitioners," we find Kenneth McLeroy (with his team of co-authors), Lawrence Green, and several other health promotion scholars (such as Minkler, 1989, 1999; Simons-Morton, Simons-Morton, Parcel, & Bunker, 1988; Steckler & Goodman, 1989; Wallerstein, Sanchez-Merki, & Dow, 1997) calling for the use of ecological and systems-science models. In the now-classic article published in 1988, McLeroy et al. proposed an "ecological model for health promotion which focuses attention on both individual *and* social environmental factors" as elements affecting human health and health behaviors. Because ecological models take into account individual level factors alongside community, or policy-level factors, they are also known as multilevel models or multilevel approaches to health promotion. According to McLeroy et al. (1998), the model

> addresses the importance of interventions directed at changing interpersonal, organizational, community, and public policy factors which support and maintain unhealthy behaviors. The model assumes that appropriate changes in the social environment will produce changes in individuals, and that the support of individuals in the population is essential for implementing environmental changes. (p. 351)

In 2008, the *American Journal of Health Promotion* published an assessment of the ecological approach in health promotion titled "The Ecological Approach in Health Promotion Programs: A Decade Later" (Kok et al., 2008). In this assessment, the authors reviewed one particular ecological approach proposed in 1996 by Lucie Richard and colleagues (Richard, Potvin, Kishchuk, Prlic, & Green, 1996). Kok and his colleagues interviewed 43 coordinators of 47 programs implemented in the United States and in The Netherlands. Based on their findings, they concluded optimistically that "health promotion practice may have changed": They found many of the programs evaluated were multilevel (with an average of 2.15 levels being targeted by each program) and aimed at promoting changes within organizations (the preferred target for change), followed by changes in policy and in communities.

While small signs of change in health promotion's individual-level focus begin to appear, in 2006, Lawrence Green and a host of authors publishing in the *American Journal of Public Health* (2006, vol. 96) called for the application of *systems science* to health promotion. These authors believe systems science:

1. Has the tools to examine numerous mediator and moderator variables.
2. Takes into account the dynamic synergy embedded among the multiple factors affecting health behaviors.
3. Assumes that complex adaptive systems (such as a human or animal population groups) can self-organize and find order within chaos (we discuss systems science and complex adaptive systems in a bit more detail in the Chapter 7).

For Green (2006),

> The social and behavioral sciences continue to be *falling short in the theories* and methods they bring to the systems needs identified by public health today. They

have enriched epidemiological understanding of causation with their inductive methods, and they have strengthened interventions by filling the gaps in evidence-based best practices with theory. *Most of their methods and theories, however, dominated as they have been by psychology, have not dealt adequately with the broader ecological understanding of causal webs and systems interventions that we seek today.* (p. 407, emphasis mine)

What exactly is systems science? In Chapter 7, we deal with nonlinear theories, and you will become more familiar with systems science. For now, it suffices to know this brief definition: Systems science or complexity science concerns itself with the study of complex adaptive systems, that is, self-organizing phenomena whose behavior is conditioned and constrained by their environments (Blackman, 2000).

There is no doubt about it: Public health in the United States (yes, there are differences in public health approaches in other countries) faces a dire need for professionals (such as you) to develop their theoretical thinking in terms of dynamic interactions among the multiple variables affecting people's health. Public health in the United States finds itself still significantly "hooked" on individual-level approaches to health and disease. A glaring example of how difficult it seems to pull away from a person-centered worldview, even when attempts are made to incorporate other nonindividual levels, may be found at the very beginning of the *Healthy People 2010* document: the "bible" for North American health promoters. When presenting and discussing Goal 1: *Increase Quality and Years of Healthy Life*, authors have this to say under the subheading *Achieving a Longer and Healthier Life—the Healthy People Perspective* (U.S. Department of Health and Human Services, 2000):

> Healthy People 2010 seeks to increase life expectancy and quality of life over the next 10 years by helping individuals gain the knowledge, motivation, and opportunities they need to make informed decisions about their health. At the same time, Healthy People 2010 encourages local and State leaders to develop communitywide and statewide efforts that promote healthy behaviors, create healthy environments, and increase access to high-quality health care. Because individual and community health are virtually inseparable, both the individual and the community need to do their parts to increase life expectancy and improve quality of life. (p. 10)

Granted, the report does mention the inextricable link between individuals' and communities' health; nevertheless, notice which point authors made *first*; upfront: that people's health stems from informed decisions, and that people arrive at these informed decisions through knowledge, motivation, and opportunities.

Such a bias has come at a high cost, however, for the effectiveness of individual-level approaches has not been impressive. A good example is smoking. Despite countless efforts to prevent and eliminate smoking behaviors, results have been unimpressive. In a recent systematic review and meta-analysis of the literature on maternal smoking during pregnancy and child overweight, the authors declare outright:

> Despite decades of research, press, counter-advertising, and litigation regarding its adverse effects, tobacco use remains a major cause of preventable morbidity and mortality world-wide. Although fewer women in the US and Britain now smoke than in past decades, an increasing number of teenage girls are initiating smoking, and smoking rates are declining less rapidly among women than among men, so cigarette smoking remains common among women who are of childbearing age, pregnant, or breast-feeding. In the developing world, a small but rapidly expanding proportion of women smoke. (Oken, Levitan, & Gillman, 2008, p. 201)

While this example puts the spotlight on smoking, similar "mixed" discouraging findings—ones showing improvements for one population group and setbacks among other groups—can be found for most other risky behaviors.

Given the complexities inherent in maintaining and promoting the well-being of entire populations, given the impact of globalization on people's health worldwide, and given the tighter and paradoxically wider networks in which people find themselves embedded, theoretical thinking in public health cannot afford to maintain a narrow, reductionist emphasis on individual-level influences on health (Tesh, 1981). It is up to you and your colleagues to promote a shift in thinking away from individual-level factors to systems-related factors. It is up to you to help turn this ship around. It's a big ship, and various attempts have historically been made to turn it around (Robertson & Minkler, 1994). Nonetheless, it is definitely *your* time to contribute to making this shift in theoretical thinking "stick."

"And just *how* do we turn this ship around?" you ask. This "journey of a thousand miles" begins with two basic steps: Step 1, *refusing* to research health-related phenomena and to implement public health interventions focusing exclusively on personal factors. One does not require extensive expertise in ecological models or systems-type theories to do this: Common-sense thinking already points to multiple factors within human environments that may impact health behaviors and decision making. Begin the healthy habit of bringing in at least one or two non–person-centered factors into your research or practice every time you face a new chance to push for prevention or to inquire into a puzzling issue. Step 2 entails beginning the process of familiarizing yourself with those theories that discuss factors *other than* intrapersonal ones. Table 5–1 lists a few of those that have, in fact, been used in health promotion. Start there: Search for studies that have used or discussed these theories. Learn about them. Teach your colleagues about them. Write about them. Expand your theoretical horizon; spread the word.

SUGGESTIONS FOR PRACTICING THEORETICAL THINKING

1. Conduct your own brief review of the literature: Go through the most recent journal articles you have read, and pencil in (or add a comment to an electronic file) the level of theory each article reports. Check your findings against what you just read in this chapter: Have most of your research reports focused on individual-level theories? If not, what level *did* they focus on? What might explain the discrepancy between your readings and what I presented in this chapter? Discuss your findings with a colleague.

2. Think about the study you're working on right now: Which levels of theories are being used? If the study focuses heavily on individual-level factors, how can the study be adapted to examine other levels of factors? Can an ecological model be applied to your study? If not, why not?

3. How can you help "turn this ship around," as I stated in this chapter? What are some action steps you can take to broaden your theoretical horizons and move away from an exclusive focus on individual-level factors?

4. What have *you* been blinded to by focusing so much on individual-level theories? Are you now able to see some of these elements you couldn't see before? Discuss this new awareness with a colleague or a mentor. Ask them about *their* experience of "seeing" and "not seeing" based on their theoretical lenses.

REFERENCES

Becker, M. H. (1986). The tyranny of health promotion. *Public Health Reviews, 14*, 15–23.

Blackman, T. (2000). Complexity theory. In G. Browning, A. Halcli, & F. Webster (Eds.), *Understanding Contemporary Society: Theories of the Present* (pp. 139–150). London: Sage Publications.

Buchanan, D. R. (2000). *An Ethic for Health Promotion: Rethinking the Sources of Human Well-Being.* New York: Oxford University Press.

Edberg, M. (2007). *Social and Behavioral Theory in Public Health.* Sudbury, MA: Jones and Bartlett Publishers.

Green, L. W. (2006). Public health asks of systems science: to advance our evidence-based practice, can you help us get more practice-based evidence? *American Journal of Public Health, 96,* 406–409.

Hancock, T. (1991). *Public Policies for Healthy Cities: Involving the Policy Makers.* Indianapolis: Indiana University School of Nursing and Institute of Action Research for Community Health.

Kok, G., Gottlieb, N. H., Commers, M., & Smerecnik, C. (2008). The ecological approach in health promotion programs: A decade later. *American Journal of Health Promotion, 22*(6), 437–447.

McLeroy, K. R., Bibeau, D., Steckler, A., & Glanz, K. (1988). An ecological perspective on health promotion programs. *Health Education Quarterly, 15*(4), 351–377.

Minkler, M. (1989). Health education, health promotion and the open society: an historical perspective. *Health Education Quarterly, 16*(1), 17–30.

Minkler, M. (1999). Personal responsibility for health? A review of the arguments and the evidence at century's end. *Health Education & Behavior, 26*(1), 121–140.

Oken, E., Levitan, E. B., & Gillman, M. W. (2008). Maternal smoking during pregnancy and child overweight: systematic review and meta-analysis. *International Journal of Obesity, 32,* 201–210.

Padilla, M. B., Hirsch, J. S., Munoz-Laboy, M., Sember, R. E., & Parkers, R. G. (Eds.). (2008). *Love and Globalization: Transformations of Intimacy in the Contemporary World.* Nashville, TN: Vanderbilt University Press.

Richard, L., Potvin, L., Kishchuk, N., Prlic, H., & Green, L. W. (1996). Assessment of the integration of the ecological approach in health promotion programs. *American Journal of Health Promotion, 10*(4), 318–328.

Robertson, A., & Minkler, M. (1994). New Health Promotion Movement: A Critical Examination. *Health Education Quarterly, 21*(3), 295–312.

Sallis, J. F., & Owen, N. (2002). Ecological Models of Health Behavior. In K. Glanz, B. K. Rimer & F. M. Lewis (Eds.), *Health Behavior and Health Education: Theory, Research, and Practice* (3rd ed., pp. 462–484). San Francisco: Jossey-Bass.

Silvia, P. J. (2007). *How to Write a Lot: A Practical Guide to Productive Academic Writing.* Washington, DC: American Psychological Association.

Simons-Morton, D. G., Simons-Morton, B. G., Parcel, G. S., & Bunker, J. F. (1988). Influencing personal and environmental conditions for community health: a multilevel intervention model. *Family and Community Health, 11*(2), 25–35.

Steckler, A., & Goodman, R. M. (1989). How to institutionalize health promotion programs. *American Journal of Health Promotion, 3*(4), 34–44.

Tesh, S. (1981). Disease causality and politics. *Journal of health Politics, Policy and Law, 6*(3), 369–390.

U.S. Department of Health and Human Services. (2000). *Healthy People 2010: Understanding and Improving Health.* Washington, DC: U.S. Department of Health and Human Services, Government Printing Office.

Wallerstein, N., Sanchez-Merki, V., & Dow, L. (1997). Feirian praxis in health education and community organizing: A case study of an adolescent prevention program. In M. Minkler (Ed.), *Community Organizing & Community Building for Health* (pp. 195–211). New Brunswick, NJ: Rutgers University Press.

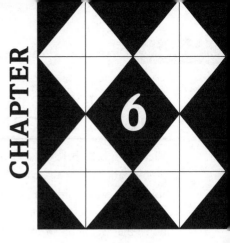

Pattern 2: Undue Emphasis on Rationality: What's Love Got to Do With It?

Learning Objectives

When you finish reading this chapter, you will be able to:

1. Identify the difficulties in approaching behavior exclusively from a cognitive, rational perspective.
2. Characterize value-expectancy and rational choice theories and their basic assumptions.
3. Characterize dual process theories.
4. Identify advantages to including affect-type constructs in health promotion theories focusing on individual-level factors.
5. Discuss why it might be in the best interest of health promotion to shift its current focus on individuals' knowledge and motivation for informed decisions to a focus on self-knowledge, awareness, life purpose, solidarity, compassion, and social justice.

VALUE-EXPECTANCY AND RATIONAL CHOICE THEORIES

Viewing health behaviors as influenced primarily by intrapersonal factors is problematic, as we've discussed in the previous chapter, but individual-level variables—we can't avoid acknowledging this—are important characters in any health promotion story. After all, it is the health of *people* (as individuals or as populations) that we, public health professionals, are interested in promoting. As stated in the Glanz book (Glanz, Rimer, & Viswanath, 2008)

> Individuals are one of the essential units of health education and health behavior theory, research, and practice. This does not mean that the individual is the only or necessarily the most important unit of intervention. But all other units, whether they are groups, organizations, worksites, communities, or larger units, are composed of individuals. (p. 41)

In Chapter 5, I concluded there is a dire need for health promoters (especially public health researchers/scholars) to shift their thinking away from individual-centered theories to more ecological or multilevel sets of explanations for health behaviors. I do not come to this conclusion lightly: I am very well aware that for some of you the mere thought of moving away from intrapersonal theories may lead you to experience withdrawal-type symptoms such as light-headedness, tremors, and anxiety. Such is the level of addiction to individual-focused theories our profession has enjoyed over the past several decades.

Even if philosophically (or, perhaps, physiologically) you find yourself unwilling to give up these individual-level explanations for health and illness, you must concede one point: The individual-level theories we have used for so many years in health promotion do not necessarily constitute the *best theories* to explain people's health-related decisions and behavior. Agree? Well, maybe not yet, but bear with me.

Here's a scenario to help you understand where I'm going with this: If you and I were having a conversation about exercise, we might talk about how we both struggle to fit exercise into our extremely busy routines (obviously, if you were an exercise aficionado we wouldn't even be having this conversation!). Oh, we *know* the value that regular exercise offers to our health, longevity, and well-being; after all, we're public health people! Yet, like many others, we struggle with trying to make exercise a priority among countless other priorities: our studies, our deadlines, our time for rest and recreation, our families and friends (not, necessarily, in this order). I am not sure about what you would say, but along with the difficulties in fitting exercise into *my* daily schedule, I would also tell you that I don't particularly *like* to exercise. I will not be terribly upset if I have to give up today's exercise session because something more pleasurable came along (a meeting with an old friend over a gourmet cup of coffee, for instance). But don't I *believe* that exercise is better for me than a super-sized dose of caffeine and dietary fat? Yes, I do believe it. . . and don't I *expect* that over time the benefits of exercise outweigh its costs and that exercise can help keep me out of a nursing home in my old age? Yes. Expect that, too. . . yet, give me the coffee-and-friend option and I'll skip exercise every time, guaranteed!

So, what is going on, here? If you were the health educator trying to help me stick to my exercise routine, what theoretical framework would you invoke to try to understand (and change) my behavior? First, you may be thinking: "I don't even need a theory to deal with that! It's easy: All I have to do is help her see the *discrepancy* in her thinking—help her see how her thinking is irrational and how she's not acting according to what she believes!" In thinking this way, you completely ignore how attracted to my discrepancies and "irrational" thinking I really am. As Epstein (1994) aptly puts it, ". . . even when people know their thinking is irrational, they often find it more compelling than their rational reasoning" (p. 712).

You might also be thinking: "All I have to do is to help this person learn to *like* exercise and to figure out how to make it her number one priority!" Okay . . . and how does one help another to *like* something they inherently dislike? How does one help someone to value something they never valued before to the point of valuing it more than other things? What factors are at play, here: a person's beliefs, outcome expectations, attitudes, perceptions of risk, perceptions of environmental barriers? What?

Well, herein resides a major difficulty underlying our use of the individual-level theories we have chosen to employ in health promotion: Most (if not all) of these theories are *value-expectancy theories*, or *rational choice theories*. Here is how Janz, Champion, and Strecher (2008) define value-expectancy theories:

> Cognitive theorists [as compared to behaviorists] . . . emphasize the role of subjective hypotheses and expectations held by the subject. . . . In this perspective, behavior is a function of the subjective *value* of an outcome and of the subjective probability, or *expectation*, that a particular action will achieve that outcome. . . . Such formulations are generally termed *value-expectancy* theories. Mental processes such as thinking, reasoning, hypothesizing, or expecting are critical components of all cognitive theories. (pp. 46–47)

Similarly, rational choice theories define human behavior as resulting from calculated reasoning. Author John Scott (2000) describes rational choice theories this way:

> Basic to all forms of rational choice theory is the assumption that complex social phenomena can be explained in terms of the elementary individual actions of which they are composed. This standpoint [is] called methodological individualism. . . . In rational choice theories, individuals are seen as motivated by the wants or goals that express their "preferences." They act within specific, given constraints and on the basis of the information that they have about the conditions under which they are acting. At its simplest, the relationship between preferences and constraints can be seen in the purely *technical* terms of the relationship of a means to an end. As it is not possible for individuals to achieve all of the various things that they want, they must also make choices in relation to both their goals and the means for attaining these goals. Rational choice theories hold that individuals must anticipate the outcomes of alternative courses of action and calculate that which will be best for them. Rational individuals choose the alternative that is likely to give them the greatest satisfaction. (pp. 127–128)

Value-expectancy or rational choice theories ground themselves on a couple of potentially problematic assumptions. First, that our decision making and behavior are determined for the most part by our cognitions, our reasoning. Second, that behind every one of our behaviors lies a checks-and-balances calculation, a risk-and-benefits assessment. It is based on a benefits-to-risk ratio that we make health behavior decisions, according to these theories. We calculate the costs and weigh the beneficial outcomes, and if the benefits outweigh the costs, we'll engage in the behavior (Janz et al., 2002). Resnicow and Page (2008) summarize this point quite well:

> Across the dominant theoretical models used by researchers and practitioners, the key determinants of behavior typically involve some variation of knowledge, attitude, belief, self-efficacy, and intention. Change is usually conceptualized as rational and as a deterministic process in which individuals obtain information, consider pros and cons, make a behavioral decision, and then plan a course of action. An implicit assumption within this perspective is that the change process is largely under conscious control. (p. 1382)

Here is the problem, however: Cognitive theories of the value-expectancy or rational choice type prove inadequate to explain why I would gladly give up an exercise session to meet a friend over a nice cup of coffee. But *why* are the theories inadequate?

The simple answer is this: because many of our behavioral choices are *not* driven by rationality, or by cognitive forces, and most of our health behavior decisions are *not* made by applying a checks-and-balances strategy. Our behaviors are driven by emotions, desires, habits, likes and dislikes, biological imperatives, and even by emotions and memories buried deep in our subconscious minds (or in our bodies; as most psychoneuroimmunologists would say: our body *is* our subconscious) (see Pert & Marriott, 2006).

Scholars from ancient wisdom literatures (such as the Bible, the Koran, and Buddhist and Hindu writings) would say we make most of our decisions with our *hearts*, not our *heads*; nevertheless, very few, if any of the theories you saw listed in Table 4–2 (in Chapter 4) will take the "heart" into consideration. It is only recently that psychological theories have begun (or, some scholars would argue, have returned to) paying attention to *affect* as an important determinant of decision making.

As David Buchanan (2000) suggests, a host of other factors usually come into play in decision making; yet similar to what happens with *affect*, health promotion theories simply ignore them:

> In Bandura's model [Social Cognitive Theory; Self-Efficacy Theory], people do not evaluate choices on the basis of a principled understanding of right and wrong, or considerations of duty and obligation, or out of reverent obedience to religious authority, or through reflection upon which ways of life might be more courageous, ennobling, or worthy, but only on the basis of their "pleasant associations" [seeking pleasure] or "aversive consequences" [avoiding pain]. (p. 74)

Which of the dominant theories we identified in Chapter 4 include courage, emotions, or subconscious factors in its set of constructs? Simpler yet, when was the last time you came across fear, anxiety, passion, or even sexual arousal as parts of models attempting to explain people's decisions to get genetic testing, to engage in a rigorous exercise program, or to use protection when having sex?[1]

---

[1] To be fair, Social Cognitive Theory includes "emotional arousal" as an important variable affecting whether people will learn a specific behavior and/or develop self-efficacy (or confidence) to perform the behavior. Yet emotional arousal is not one of the factors health educators remember *first* when asked to list the most important variables addressed by Social Cognitive Theory. Outcome expectations, expectancies, observational learning, and self-efficacy are the most commonly recalled and the most commonly addressed factors (in health promotion interventions/programs).

DUAL PROCESS THEORIES—BEYOND RATIONALITY

Interestingly enough, if you step outside public health, and observe the theoretical landscape in other fields such as economy (e.g., consumer behavior studies), political science (voting behaviors), and psychology itself, you will encounter quite a bit more options for theoretically understanding human behaviors. Guess what scholars in these fields are now saying? Yes, human behaviors, choices, and decisions are *not exclusively governed* by rationality or cognitive factors.

Here are some examples of such thinking in these fields. In psychology, theories describing how people process information have begun to develop as "dual process theories" (Chaiken & Trope, 1999). According to Steven A. Sloman, writing in 1996, the debate between scholars whether humans process information in an exclusively cognitive manner (calculating risks and benefits) or in an "emotional" manner (acting on "gut" feelings, responding to fears, or reacting to traumatic past experiences) "has raged (again) in cognitive psychology for almost a decade now" (Sloman, 1996). The story these "dual process theories" tell about how people deal with information includes two different elements: affective and cognitive. The theories themselves vary on a continuum in terms of how much emphasis is placed on the cognitive or the affective elements. Nonetheless, these theories insist the two are continually interacting and influence different decisions in different ways. As you can see, these theories present a landscape that has gradually moved away from an exclusive emphasis on rationality or cognition to include affect (emotions) (Gelder, De Vries, & Pligt, 2009).

Dual-process theories have recently been applied to the study of how people handle information about *risk* (something we, in public health, are quite interested in influencing). In this regard, I recall reading and reviewing a book called *Sex and Sexuality: Risk and Relationships in the Age of AIDS* (Goodson, 1999). The book reported a qualitative study of young college students and how they perceived and handled the risk of becoming HIV positive and developing AIDS when engaging in casual sexual relationships. I believe the most intriguing and engaging finding in that study related to how these students viewed the risk of becoming infected: The risk was never absolute (i.e., you have several sexual partners, you have a higher risk of contracting HIV). It was always *relative*: For many study participants, the risk of contracting HIV might be *smaller than* the risk of emotional pain resulting from a breakup of the relationship. Relationships could be affected by one partner's insistence in taking protective measures to avoid the risk of contracting HIV; therefore, study participants managed risk more in an affective manner than in a calculated manner. Dual-process theories take such "affective manner," the feelings surrounding the management of health risks, into account and pay serious attention to them.

Since reading that book, I have had a hard time with the way we in health promotion, public health, and medicine deal with the construct *risk*, in such cognitive, nonemotional, terms. Approaching *risk* from a purely rational, cognitive perspective has significant implications for public health and health care practices. Consider, for instance, the way public health professionals:

1. *Talk* about risk: "If you have multiple partners your risk is high of getting HIV or another sexually transmitted infection."

2. *Communicate* risk information in terms of *percentages and probabilities*: "Your genotype reveals you have a 25% chance of transmitting this defective gene to one of your biological children."

3. *Expect the public to rationally act* upon the risk information we provide: The breast cancer gene runs in your family; you should consider all possible options for preventing the cancer: a radical mastectomy, perhaps. (And before you scream how atrocious this recommendation seems, keep in mind it's not mine: several studies have examined the risks and benefits of prophylactic mastectomies for women with genetic risk for breast cancer; see, e.g., Heemskerk-Gerritsen et al., 2007; and Kasprzak et al., 2005.)

My difficulty with how we deal with risk information stems precisely from the incontrovertible fact that we present (and expect clients to deal with) risk information only in *rational* terms. We rarely, if ever, deal with the emotions embedded in giving, receiving, and processing the information.

Scholars studying a variety of human behaviors that involve decisions or choices have begun to sound the call to add *affect, emotions, or feelings* to current theoretical models. Those actively conducting research using these enhanced models have found that they outperform cognitive-based ones when explaining certain types of behaviors or decisions. Adding fuel to this fire, researchers have simultaneously begun to document the inadequate performance of cognitive-based theories in explaining and predicting behavior change.

Studying voters' preferences during elections, Wang (2008), for instance, tested two models predicting public choice of presidential candidates (before the 2004 Presidential Election in the United States): a cognitive and an affect-based model. The cognitive model focused on elements such as the important political and social issues surrounding the election and candidates' likelihood of success in dealing with those. The affect-based model included "four sets of interpersonal emotions" that study participants used to rate (or choose) the presidential candidates: admiration, contempt, envy, and pity. Participants were asked to "rate on a 5-point scale their emotional reactions to the presidential candidates Bush and Kerry" (Wang, 2008, p. 85). Not surprisingly, findings supported the notion that the affect-based model explained public choice of candidates better than the cognitive-based model (Wang, 2008).

As another example, Ariely and Loewenstein (2006) conducted a study to assess whether sexual arousal (one type of affect variable) would impact the following choices and judgments, made by a sample of young adult males (p. 88):

1. Their preferences for a wide range of sexual stimuli and activities
2. Their willingness to engage in morally questionable behaviors in order to obtain sexual gratification
3. Their willingness to engage in unsafe sex when sexually aroused

Despite an important limitation in that study—sexual arousal measures were obtained through self-report—its findings and conclusions are worthy of notice (Ariely & Loewenstein, 2006):

> Our results . . . suggest that sexual arousal acts as an amplifier of sorts. Activities that are not perceived as arousing when young males are not sexually aroused become sexually charged and attractive when they are, and those activities that are attractive even when not aroused, become more attractive under the influence of arousal. . . . Our results further suggest that . . . the increase in motivation to have sex produced by sexual arousal seems to decrease the relative importance of other considerations such as behaving ethically toward a potential sexual partner or protecting oneself against unwanted pregnancy or sexually transmitted disease. (p. 95)

The authors conclude that people's sexual choices and behaviors can alter significantly when they become sexually aroused and that attempts to influence sexual behaviors cannot rely exclusively on nonaroused reasoning and rationality (something, I believe, most of us know from personal experience).

Additional support for the notion that cognitive factors may not be the most significant forces influencing human behavior comes from a meta-analytic study conducted by Webb and Paschal in 2006. The meta-analysis assessed whether changing people's intentions leads them to change their behavior (a rather popular notion in health promotion, today). After the study, the authors concluded that

> . . . A medium-to-large change in intention (d = 0.66) engenders a small-to-medium change in behavior (d = *0.36*). Thus, intention has a significant impact on behavior, but the size of this effect is considerably smaller than correlational tests have suggested. (p. 260)

The connection, therefore, between intention and behavior, upon which several of our theories hinge and many of our interventions are built, is weaker than first believed. In fact, Webb and Paschal go as far as documenting in their analysis that in some of the studies meta-analyzed *behaviors affected intentions* (i.e., the relationship occurred in the opposite direction, from that originally proposed in most of the *intention → behavior* models).

The take-home message, therefore, is this: Many scholars studying human decision-making and specific behaviors have concluded that most decisions and behaviors are not based on rationality or reasoning alone; rather, forces such as affect, emotions, and sexual arousal have a strong influence in the decision-making process or may even constitute its main drivers.

In summary, as we observe the development and refinement of theories in fields outside public health—stating that humans process information, make decisions, and behave because they are influenced by at least two sets of forces ("one variously labeled intuitive, automatic, natural, nonverbal, narrative, and experiential, and the other analytical, deliberative, verbal, and rational"—(Epstein, 1994, p. 710)—it becomes clear that our health promotion theories are lopsided: They have only dealt with one set of factors, namely the rational set. The other, has been, thus far, conveniently ignored.

AN ALTERNATIVE

One alternative (but, surely, not the only one) to this myopic perspective is the inclusion of affect-type variables within the existing behavioral models and/or the adoption of other theories entirely (Gelder et al., 2009). Two examples of individual-level theories worth exploring and perhaps adding to the health promotion theoretical arsenal are Cognitive-Experiential Self-Theory (CEST), proposed by Epstein (1994), and the model of interpersonal behavior (MIP), developed by Triandis (1980). CEST adds *affect* to a set of cognitive factors, and the MIP adds the element of *habits*, or habitual behavior, to reasoning constructs.

Introduced in 1973, CEST explains human decision-making as consisting of two distinct, but highly overlapping processes (Epstein, 1994):

> It is assumed [in CEST] that there are two major systems by which people adapt to the world: rational and experiential. People have constructs about the self and

the world in both systems. Those in the rational system are referred to as *beliefs* and those in the experiential system as *implicit beliefs* or, alternatively, as *schemata*. The schemata . . . consist primarily of generalizations derived from emotionally significant past experience. . . . All behavior is assumed, in CEST, to be the product of the joint operation of [the] two systems. Their relative dominance is determined by various parameters, including individual differences in style of thinking and situational variables. (p. 715)

Another interesting and potentially useful framework is the model of interpersonal behavior (MIP). Proposed by Triandis in 1980, MIP is quite similar to the Theory of Reasoned Action (TRA) and Theory of Planned Behavior (TPB) because it strongly values the construct of "intention" as one of the main determinants of behavior. Also in line with the TRA and TPB, the MIP affirms the importance of having control over the behavior, along with the appropriate intentions, for the behavior to happen (don't you just *love it* when authors use acronyms, left-and-right, in a sentence?); nevertheless, the "twist" comes when MIP also emphasizes the importance of *habits* (Webb & Paschal, 2006):

. . . the MIP also postulates a second potential moderator of intention realization, namely, the extent to which the behavior is habitual. According to Triandis (1980), frequently performed behaviors are likely to come under the control of habits, and the impact of intentions on behavior is thereby reduced. (p. 250)

Habits, along with emotions, are important to recognize when public health professionals are trying to help people discard certain behaviors and adopt new ones (especially when those habits have an addiction element to them). Habitual behaviors are, at times, the most unresponsive to behavior change efforts, as we well know (Triandis, 1980).

Another alternative to consider is incorporating more of the theoretical frameworks and findings from psychoneuroimmunology, which attempts to view human beings holistically, as a mind-body-soul indivisible unit, itself a manifestation of a broader, quantum energy pattern (Chopra, 1991/2000; McTaggart, 2007; Pert, 1997). Dr. Deepak Chopra—an endocrinologist and world-renowned leader of the mind–body health movement—uses the example of heart attacks (especially those that happen at 9:00 a.m., to people who hate their jobs) to make his point regarding the inextricable link between body and mind:

At the quantum mechanical level, mind and body are united; therefore, it comes as no surprise that a deep, smoldering dissatisfaction lodged in the mind should express itself in a physical equivalent—a heart attack.

Indeed, any dissatisfaction *must* express itself physically, because all our thoughts turn into chemicals. When you are happy, chemicals in your brain travel throughout your body, telling every cell of your happiness. When they hear the message, the cells "get happy," too; that is, they begin to function more effectively by altering their own chemical processes. If you are depressed, on the other hand, the opposite happens. Your sadness is relayed chemically to each cell, causing a feeling of heartache, for example, and your immune system to grow weaker. Everything we think and do originates inside the quantum mechanical body and then bubbles up to the surface of life. (Chopra, 1991/2000, p. 140)

Not only could we be using theories that validate this body–mind unity and incorporate emotional constructs, we might, in fact, begin looking to theories that validate the multiple levels of reality in which human beings are immersed. Many scholars in the various traditions of enlightenment propose that the forces driving and influencing human behavior may be found at multiple levels of reality (not merely at multiple environmental levels, as most ecological models propose). Chopra suggests, for instance, at least three domains or levels of human existence, all of which shape and affect our everyday living, decision making, and behavior (Chopra, 2003, pp. 35–46):

1. The physical domain (the realm of the physical universe, of material and visible objects that surround us)
2. The quantum domain (the realm of information and energy; the world of the mind and all other nonvisible realities)
3. The nonlocal domain (the realm of intelligence or consciousness; "the virtual domain, the field of potential, the universal being, or nonlocal intelligence")

Even though quantum physics provides support for the existence of these domains (McTaggart, 2002, 2007), many health professionals choose to operate and understand human life strictly from a physical domain, denying the possibility that other nonphysical realities might affect human behavior and the choices people make regarding their well-being, their life trajectories, their relationships, and their physical/mental/spiritual health.

Many public health scholars and practitioners shrug and say these aspects or domains of human life are not the purview of health promotion efforts because they do not belong in the scientific realm. "We are not psychologists, or therapists, or even counselors, to delve into these dimensions," they say. Although they don't perceive themselves as psychologists, they have no qualms about borrowing heavily from psychology's theories, and about speaking the language psychologists speak, to explain behaviors in a "scientific way." Interesting inconsistency. . . .

While public health lags behind, reluctant to address the various dimensions of human life in prevention and health promotion efforts, many "pockets" of the healing professions have already welcomed restorative strategies that tap on the nonphysical domains of existence. In a cursory search, we observe substantial amounts of the therapy/treatment literature applying mindfulness techniques (such as meditation, yoga, qigong, relaxation, intentionality, visualization, and journaling) to help people manage stress, improve self-awareness, and foster intentional behavior (i.e., behavior that is not automatic, but consciously generated) (Shapiro, Carlson, Astin, & Freedman, 2006). Homeopathy, acupuncture, and chiropractic—just a few of the holistic forms of medicine available to most of us—have been putting into practice energy-based, holistic treatments that are centuries old (or thousands of years old, in the case of acupuncture) (see Eisenberg & Wright, 1995; Koch, 1995; Matchim & Armer, 2007; Praissman, 2008).

Unfortunately, we do not see such approaches in the health promotion/prevention literature. Only among those who view health promotion critically might we encounter suggestions for strategies that include the various dimensions of human life. David Buchanan—one of these critics—contends that health promoters *could consider changing* their intervention strategies: moving away from both cognitive-based factors and simple cause-and-effect formulas. From Buchanan's perspective, given the "complex portrait of life," it "makes little sense to speak of causal or independent risk factors," and health promoters should, therefore, rethink their methods for promoting health. He says, "In a different frame of mind, health promoters might think about the kinds of social practices that engender *attentiveness, mindfulness, responsive openness*" (Buchanan, 2000, p. 114).

Buchanan offers, in his book, a few (very few, in fact) examples of successful initiatives applying such practices. One of the examples he describes constitutes "true" health promotion, yet wasn't started by health care or even by health promotion professionals: Alcoholics Anonymous (AA) (Gerstein & Harwood, 1990). Describing AA's operations as "a group of people who voluntarily come together to discuss issues of common concern, meeting in open public spaces . . . [where] there are no scientists, no skilled professionals, no therapists leading the session"—Buchanan (2000) somberly concludes, regarding these and similar strategies:

> It is *this* type of practice, I believe, that holds the most promise for the future of health promotion. It is a collective cooperative human activity aimed at realizing the good for human beings through fostering *self-knowledge, autonomy, integrity, respect, responsibility, solidarity, and social action* to expand the sphere of *justice* in this world. (p. 115, emphasis mine)

Just for the sake of curiosity, compare Buchanan's previous statement with the statement under Goal 1 in the Healthy People 2010 document I transcribed in Chapter 5. I used that Healthy People 2010 statement there to illustrate the United States' continued addiction to individual-level factors. Yet that statement also spotlights the emphasis being given to rational, cognitive factors. Here's the statement (U.S. Department of Health and Human Services, 2000):

> Healthy People 2010 seeks to increase life expectancy and quality of life over the next 10 years by helping individuals gain the *knowledge, motivation,* and *opportunities* they need to make informed *decisions* about their health. (p. 10, emphasis mine)

A different practice, we propose (Buchanan and I), would move health promotion away from merely helping individuals gain knowledge, motivation, and opportunities to make informed decisions about health to helping people gain self-knowledge, awareness, life purpose, solidarity, compassion, and a sense of social justice to enhance their own, their community's, and the world's health and well-being simultaneously. It is time that health promotion became holistic, in the best sense of the term, and was perceived as a truly "alternative, complementary, and *syn*-energy based" practice.

Why isn't health promotion as a field and most of our intervention efforts then adopting holistic techniques as its *modus operandi*? After all, approaching human behavior from a holistic perspective is not an innovation that we must first try out to see if it works—as we would with any other innovation (according to Roger's Diffusion of Innovations theory) (see Rogers, 1962). It has been extensively tested, proven effective, and documented from ancient literature texts to electronic journal articles. So, what happens?

In a nutshell, the main difficulty lies in health promotion's desire to become more closely aligned with a scientific, medical model of disease prevention (Buchanan, 2000). Because health promotion has chosen to describe human health, health behaviors, prevention, and treatment as components of a scientific story (which privileges *causes* and *effects* as the main characters in the plot), all other stories considered nonscientific have no place. It doesn't matter that these other stories explain things better, have fewer negative side-effects, or promote health and social justice in more purposeful ways. The more health promotion wishes to only tell *one type* of story about health and illness, the more it will ignore all other (even potentially *better*) stories. Holistic approaches to health promotion are still perceived as standing "outside the space" of science, at the fringes of scientific thought. They are still viewed as nonvalid stories.

The main alternative here is clear: To turn this ship around, a major paradigm shift will need to occur. Privileging all dimensions of human existence will only happen in public health practice once professionals (like *you*) are willing to write, and tell, other types of stories about what constitutes an individual person, about health and disease, about the good life humans can live in community, about the life worth living, and about the value of health as a means to other, larger goals (Buchanan, 2000). It is time to consider whether *you* might want to take part in such a paradigm shifting, such a theoretical task.

SUGGESTIONS FOR PRACTICING THEORETICAL THINKING

1. Examine the research publications you have read, recently, and select those that focus on individual-level factors. See whether any of these reports showcase any of the affect-type variables discussed in this chapter.
2. Discuss with your colleagues (or mentors) what it would take to begin shifting the focus from rational-choice-type theories to dual process theories in health promotion.
3. Consider one of your research projects that focus on individual-level variables: If you haven't done so, already, could you employ a more balanced theoretical approach, one that includes both cognitive and affective variables? Share your ideas with a colleague.

REFERENCES

Ariely, D., & Loewenstein, G. (2006). The heat of the moment: the effect of sexual arousal on sexual decision making. *Journal of Behavioral Decision Making, 19,* 87–98.

Buchanan, D. R. (2000). *An Ethic for Health Promotion: Rethinking the Sources of Human Well-Being.* New York: Oxford University Press.

Chaiken, S., & Trope, Y. (Eds.). (1999). *Dual-Process Theories in Social Psychology.* New York: The Guilford Press.

Chopra, D. (1991/2000). *Perfect Health: The Complete Mind Body Guide* (Revised Edition ed.). New York: Three Rivers Press.

Chopra, D. (2003). *The Spontaneous Fulfillment of Desire: Harnessing the Infinite Power of Coincidence.* New York: Harmony Books.

Eisenberg, D., & Wright, T. L. (1995). *Encounters with Qi: Exploring Chinese Medicine.* New York: W.W. Norton & Company.

Epstein, S. (1994). Integration of the cognitive and the psychodynamic unconscious. *American Psychologist, 49*(8), 709–724.

Gelder, J.-L., De Vries, R. E., & Pligt, J. v. d. (2009). Evaluating a dual-process model of risk: affect and cognition as determinants of risky choice. *Journal of Behavioral Decision Making, 22,* 45–61.

Gerstein, D., & Harwood, H. (Eds.). (1990). *Treating Drug Problems* (Vol. I). Washington, DC: National Academy Press.

Glanz, K., Rimer, B. K., & Viswanath, K. (2008). *Health Behavior and Health Education: Theory, Research, and Practice* (4th ed.). San Francisco: Jossey-Bass.

Goodson, P. (1999). Sex and sexuality: risk and relationships in the age of aids—review. *Health Education and Behavior, 26*(5), 751–753.

Heemskerk-Gerritsen, B. A. M., Brekelmans, C. T. M., Menke-Pluymers, M. B. E., et al. (2007). Prophylactic mastectomy in BRCA1/2 mutation carriers and women at risk of hereditary breast cancer: long-term experiences at the Rotterdam Family Cancer Clinic. *Annals of Surgical Oncology, 14*(12), 3335–3344.

Janz, N. K., Champion, V. L., & Strecher, V. J. (2002). The health belief model. In K. Glanz, B. K. Rimer, & F. M. Lewis (Eds.), *Health Behavior and Health Education* (pp. 45–66). San Francisco: Jossey-Bass.

Kasprzak, L., Mesurolle, B., Tremblay, F., Galvez, M., Halwani, F., & Foulkes, W. D. (2005). Invasive breast cancer following bilateral subcutaneous mastectomy in a BRCA2 mutation carrier: a case report and review of the literature. *World Journal of Surgical Oncology, 3,* 52–58.

Koch, W. H. (1995). *Chiropractic: The Superior Alternative.* Calgary Alberta, Canada: Bayeux Arts Incorporated.

Matchim, Y., & Armer, J. M. (2007). Measuring the psychological impact of mindfulness meditation on health among patients with cancer: a literature review. *Oncology Nursing Forum, 34*(5), 1059–1066.

McTaggart, L. (2002). *The Field: The Quest For The Secret Force of the Universe.* New York: Harper Perennial.

McTaggart, L. (2007). *The Intention Experiment.* New York: Free Press.

Pert, C. B. (1997). *Molecules of Emotion: The Science behind Mind-Body Medicine.* New York: Scribner.

Pert, C. B., & Marriott, N. (2006). *Everything You Need to Know to Feel Go(o)d.* Carlsbad, CA: Hay House, Inc.

Praissman, S. (2008). Mindfulness-based stress reduction: a literature review and clinician's guide. *Journal of the American Academy of Nurse Practitioners, 20,* 212–216.

Resnicow, K., & Page, S. E. (2008). Embracing chaos and complexity: a quantum change for public health. *American Journal of Public Health, 98*(8), 1382–1389.

Rogers, E. M. (1962). *Diffusion of Innovations* (5th ed.). New York: Free Press.

Scott, J. (2000). Rational choice theory. In G. Browning, A. Halci, & F. Webster (Eds.), *Understanding Contemporary Society: Theories of the Present* (pp. 126–138). London: Sage Publications.

Shapiro, S. L., Carlson, L. E., Astin, J. A., & Freedman, B. (2006). Mechanisms of mindfulness. *Journal of Clinical Psychology, 62*(3), 373–386.

Sloman, S. A. (1996). The empirical case for two systems of reasoning. *Psychological Bulletin, 119*(1), 3–22.

Triandis, H. C. (1980). *Values, attitudes, and interpersonal behavior.* Paper presented at the Nebraska symposium of motivation, Lincoln, NE.

U.S. Department of Health and Human Services. (2000). *Healthy People 2010: Understanding and Improving Health.* Washington, DC: U.S. Department of Health and Human Services, Government Printing Office.

Wang, X. T. (2008). Decision heuristics as predictors of public choice. *Journal of Behavioral Decision Making, 21,* 77–89.

Webb, T. L., & Paschal, S. (2006). Does changing behavioral intentions engender behavior change? A meta-analysis of the experimental evidence? *Psychological Bulletin, 132*(2), 249–268.

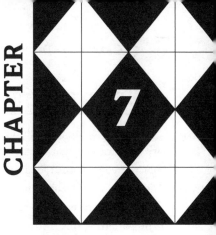

CHAPTER 7

Pattern 3: Deliberate Privileging of Linearity: The Whole or the Sum of the Parts?

Learning Objectives

When you finish reading this chapter, you will be able to:

1. Compare the main characteristics of linear and nonlinear theories.
2. Identify the reasons why the study of human behavior might benefit from a nonlinear perspective.
3. Define Complex Adaptive Systems, and identify examples of health-related Complex Adaptive Systems.
4. Propose an alternative to health promotion's deliberate focus on linear theories.
5. Point to at least two limitations inherent in studying human behavior from a complexity science perspective.

LINEAR THEORIES

While journeying through the current theoretical landscape in health promotion we have learned that the theories most frequently deployed in our research and practice come with at least two problematic patterns: (1) an exaggerated focus on individual-level factors and (2) a concentrated attention on cognitive variables. The trip doesn't end here, however. There is still one important pattern to explore. The pattern is this: Most of the theories you saw listed in Table 4–2 are *linear theories*.

One way to understand the notion of linear theories is to think about the traditional stories told by scientists regarding the natural and the social world(s). These stories—concocted since the early beginnings of the natural sciences (think physics and astronomy, for instance)—have been profoundly influenced by the work of Sir Isaac Newton; so influenced, in fact, that when scientists think about "linearity," or "linear theories," they often refer to them as "Newtonian theories or models."

Newton had a special interest in the movement of objects (especially planets' orbits) and the development of machines. His approach to learning about the world consisted of breaking down a large complex entity, such as the solar system for instance, into its constituent parts. Observing the individual parts and learning about each one allowed him to understand and explain the entire system. His approach carried over to machines: To understand how a certain machine works—for example, a clock—all one needed to do, from Newton's point of view, was to take it apart and learn about its smaller pieces. After learning all about each individual piece, one could understand the whole: The whole was equal to the sum of its parts.

This *"the whole is equal to the sum of the parts"* Newtonian approach and its language (mathematics) remained the dominant theme within the stories told by science until very recently. This reign lasted for quite a long time, in fact, since Sir Isaac Newton was alive and publishing his work during the late 17th and early 18th centuries. His mechanistic approach to scientific learning influenced even the study of human anatomy and physiology. We owe the notion that our bodies function as "perfectly oiled machines" to Sir Isaac Newton himself. Cooper and Geyer (2008) provide a nice summary of this history and its impact on social sciences and public health:

> The current mainstream traditional framework [for health promotion and care] emerged out of the physical sciences in the 17th, 18th and 19th centuries. Founded on the work of Newton, Descartes and many others, it assumed that

the physical world acted like a giant mechanical clock and ran according to fundamental and immutable physical laws. This framework emphasized the four basic rules of predictability, causality, reductionism and determinism.

These rules have been tremendously powerful and acted as the foundation of many of the developments of the industrial revolution and the basic institutional structure for modern universities and hospitals. Unsurprisingly, the human and social sciences were not unaffected by these developments. Though challenged from a variety of perspectives, this orderly, linear framework remains the mainstream foundation of the human and social sciences to this day. (pp. 177–178)

So it is that even psychology, sociology, and other sciences from which public health borrows its theories have emphasized a linear perspective when studying human behavior and social phenomena. Most of the theories listed in Table 4–2 concern themselves with predicting health behaviors, identifying their causes, reducing the large plethora of causes to a manageable few, and proposing that such causal mechanisms can, in fact, be predicted, influenced, and changed according to the public health agenda at that historical moment.

Yet, over time, Newtonian linear approaches—despite their "mainstream" status—began to prove inadequate when it came to explaining certain phenomena, when, as Tim Blackman (2000) wisely stated, "reality demand[ed] it, which [was] surprisingly often" (p. 143). Zimmerman (2000a) explains it well:

The Newtonian perspective assumes that all can be explained by the careful examination of the parts. Yet that does not work for many aspects of human behavior. We have all experienced situations in which the whole is not the sum of the parts—where we cannot explain the outcomes of a situation by studying the individual elements. For example, when a natural disaster strikes a community, we have seen spontaneous organization where there is no obvious leader, controller or designer. In these contexts, we find groups of people create outcomes and have impacts which are far greater than would have been predicted by summing up the resources and skills available with the group. In these cases, there is self-organization in which outcomes emerge which are highly dependent on the relationships and context rather than merely the parts. (p. 1)

COMPLEXITY THEORIES

In health promotion, we study human behavior. Human behavior rarely occurs in isolation. It results from many *interactions*; for we, humans, find ourselves embedded in a variety of different contexts, different systems (families, communities, schools, neighborhoods, clubs, and professional groups). Even when it occurs in isolation (think perhaps of a hermit living in a solitary cabin in the woods), human behavior is constantly changing or adapting and is, itself, the result of the dynamic interaction of a large number of intrapersonal motivators or forces (from biological to self-actualization needs, for instance). Don't we always say that the only "constant" in human life is "change"? Linear theories cannot account for constant change, for the outcomes resulting from complex relationships, and for the unpredictability inherent in human behavior, because human behavior rarely—if ever—results from the sum of the individual forces that drive it or lends itself to reliable prediction (Cooper & Geyer, 2008; Resnicow & Page, 2008):

> Human beings are the most complex of all [living beings and living systems] because not only are we physical and biologically complex systems, but we have the conscious capacity to interpret, evaluate and create narratives about our lives, societies and histories that affect our actions, understanding and development. . . . From this perspective, the core rules for understanding human complexity and complex systems are very different from those of the orderly framework of [linear theories]. (Cooper & Geyer, 2008, p. 178)

Also referred to as *complexity theories, complexity science, systems science, dynamic systems theories* and, more popularly, *chaos theory* (but beware: these terms are not exact synonyms), nonlinear theories concern themselves with systems exhibiting complex behaviors or characteristics. A simple definition of nonlinear theories then is this: Nonlinear theories study *complex adaptive systems*, the relationship patterns within these systems, how they sustain themselves, how they self-organize, and how outcomes emerge (Zimmerman, Lindberg, & Plsek 1998).

Complex Adaptive Systems

What are complex adaptive systems, this central tenet of nonlinear theories? Well, let's break the phrase apart, following Zimmerman, Lindberg, and Plsek's (1998) suggestion: a "system" refers to a set of connected or interdependent "things" (or agents, such as persons, molecules, organizations, or species). Another way to define "systems" is to describe them as "nested bundles of shared information within networks of information exchanges" (Blackman, 2000, p. 144). The term "adaptive" refers to the capacity to change, the ability to learn from experience; and the term "complex" implies diversity, or a large number of connections among a variety of elements; therefore, Complex Adaptive Systems (CASs) consist of a set of interacting elements that are able to change and adapt in multiple ways (Zimmerman, Lindberg, & Plsek, 1998).

Unfortunately, it is beyond the scope of this chapter to provide a detailed description of complexity theories, but I would encourage you to read and become more familiar with them. For an excellent treatment of chaos theory (one type of nonlinear theory, showcased in the book and movie *Jurassic Park*) and how it emerged in various fields of science (almost simultaneously, which is a fascinating story in itself!), I highly recommend you read the book *Chaos*, by James Gleick (1987). For now, it is enough to keep in mind that nonlinear, complex systems theories propose the following about CASs:

1. The whole is much more than the sum of its parts.
2. CASs consist of other CASs: Each individual agent in a CAS is itself a CAS.
3. The agents in a CAS evolve with the CAS to which they belong.
4. Diversity is *necessary* for the sustainability of a CAS. A decrease in diversity reduces the potential for future adaptations; diversity is key to innovation and long term viability of a CAS.
5. CASs exhibit distributed control rather than centralized control (i.e., control is distributed throughout the system vs. a "command center"). This means that the outcomes of a CAS emerge from a process of self-organization rather than being designed and controlled externally or by a centralized body.
6. CASs are nonlinear systems: The size of the outcome may not be correlated to the size of the input.
7. CASs exhibit sensitive dependence to initial conditions (also known as "the butterfly effect"); they are history dependent.
8. CASs are naturally drawn to attractors. The attractor is a pattern or area that draws the energy of the system to it.
9. CASs manifest unpredictable behavior.
10. In a CAS, order underlies even what appears to be disordered or chaotic.

This is adapted from Zimmerman, Lindberg, and Plsek (pp. 8–13, 1998). I highly recommend this source for additional information on complex systems theories.

Can you think of a few examples of complex adaptive systems based on these characteristics? Imagine ecosystems in nature. Think of weather systems. Visualize kids playing in a kindergarten playground. Think of viruses multiplying within a living host. Think of the human body, neural connections in the human brain, the development of a human fetus, human relationships, and communities. All of these constitute examples of complex adaptive systems. Repeating what we said previously, Newtonian theories prove themselves inadequate to study CASs because linear approaches cannot account for the following:

1. The dynamic changes or adaptations occurring within the system
2. The interactions among the elements of the system
3. The interactions among various systems

Linear Versus Dynamic Approaches to Human Reality

Here's an example that may help you understand the differences between a linear and a nonlinear approach to human reality, a bit better: Think of a school district that finds itself in trouble. The district suffers from chronic low academic performance, strong achievement disparities among its students, and low morale. Administrators or policy makers responsible for dealing with the problems, who think in a linear fashion, will identify one or more causes for these problems. Let's suppose they conclude that the lack of resources, specifically the lack of money and appropriate educational technology are the two most important reasons the school district is floundering. If lack of money and technology appear to *cause* the problems in that school district, linear logic will propose that more money and more technology will lead to higher performance, fewer achievement disparities, and improved morale. The solution? Invest more resources in that school district. Right? Right, from a linear thinking perspective it sounds perfectly reasonable.

Yet, after resources are pumped into the system, administrators find the impact of their investment in more money and more technology has produced limited, if not negligible results: Performance improved only slightly. Disparities are actually more pronounced, and the morale is so-so. . . . What happened? What went wrong? Why didn't things turn out as expected? After all, the causes of the problem were identified and dealt with, weren't they? Administrators knew what caused the problems; they had a plan to "correct" the causes. Why didn't the effects follow suit?

Nonlinear theories focus on these apparent "anomalies" (which are only "anomalies" from a linear perspective, of course). Quite often, a nonlinear perspective only emerges when things don't quite "work" in a linear way. In the case of the troubled school district, a nonlinear-thinking consultant would have detected that the cultural and personal dynamics of the leaders in that district, coupled with how these leaders dealt with (or related to) the teachers, staff, students, and the community at large was negatively impacting all interpersonal relationships in that district. Instead of "throwing money" at the problem, nonlinear thinkers might suggest bringing in one or more new leaders who could foster positive communication and relationships among members in the district. Perhaps all it might take is changing one or a couple of people; the resulting change in dynamics is unpredictable and therefore full of possibilities! Changing one agent in the system and providing room for the system to self-organize might have been the only minor alterations required to turn that school district around, with impressive and unexpected results.

While this school district example may help us understand how linear and nonlinear approaches might look in the real world, a metaphor might help us appreciate the unique characteristics of nonlinearity. So here is an image that might help you see the essential, qualitative difference between linear and nonlinear ways of thinking: a picture puzzle. Think of linear and nonlinear theories as different types of puzzles, with rather distinct characteristics. When we solve a linear jigsaw puzzle, we see the final picture only after putting the pieces together in a specific way. Usually, there is only *one* way of joining the pieces, and the final fitting yields only a *single* image. The image represents the agglomeration of all the tiny pieces (sometimes thousands!) forming the puzzle. If it happens that one or more pieces are missing, the final picture will be incomplete, and the missing information will be evident.

Yet other types of puzzles, for instance, holographic puzzles (or nonlinear puzzles), behave quite uniquely because holograms display very interesting properties. Here's one of them: While only a single image emerges from the linear puzzle, the image emerging from a holographic puzzle changes according to the perspective from which the viewer sees the pieces. Looked at from one direction, viewers see image A (for instance, a bowl of fruit). Seen from another direction, viewers see image B (for example, the same bowl of fruit, now with a hand grabbing one of the apples inside the bowl).

Not only can various images emerge from a single holographic medium, these images share another interesting property (Lincoln & Guba, 1985):

> If a normal recording or a normal film were damaged in some way—for instance, through the loss of some portion of the whole—then that same portion of information would also be lost. If a section of sound tape is cut out for 18 minutes, say, those 18 minutes are forever gone. Or if the image of a man is cropped out of a negative of a group picture, the association of that man with that group is forever destroyed. But holographs have the property that, *even if* large portions of the recorded interference patterns are lost, the remaining pieces, no matter how tiny, will all have complete information and will be able

to reproduce the original image in its entirety (and in three dimensions!). Every piece of a system has complete information about the whole. . . . *Thus, while the whole is more than the sum of its parts, each part contains the whole within itself.* (p. 53, emphasis mine)

When we compare linear and nonlinear theories to these different types of puzzles, we begin to notice that linear theories strive to produce a single, one-faceted, and static explanation of human behavior (e.g., poor nutrition leads to obesity). Nonlinear theories—by looking at relationships, interactions, and the contexts for human behavior—provide multiple explanations, or multiple images, of a given phenomenon (poor nutrition, in this perspective, requires interaction with other intrapersonal and environmental factors to actually cause obesity). Moreover, nonlinear theories observe human behavior not merely as resulting from multiple contextual forces, but also as a force itself, influencing (and, to an extent, reproducing in itself) all other elements of the system.

Linear Versus Nonlinear Data Analyses

Where public health's overemphasis on linearity becomes strikingly visible is in the analysis of quantitative data from empirical studies of health issues. Most of the statistical analyses employed presuppose a linear relationship between variables: More of X is associated with more of Y in a positive or direct relationship; more of X is associated with less of Y in an inverse or negative relationship. Even the more sophisticated data analyses techniques, which assume complex interactions among many factors (more closely resembling the complexities found in human realities; see Buhi, Goodson, & Neilands, 2007), even these techniques presuppose a positive or negative relationship among variables, but always a linear one.

When we study multiple regression in statistics courses, for instance, we learn that the purpose of the analysis is to fit a straight line across many data points so the line sits as closely as possible to these points. Students find themselves baffled when they see a graph such as the one in Figure 7–1A and hear from their instructors that the goal is to find the best fitting straight line that can represent all (or most) of those data points. . . . Huh? A straight line to represent this apparent "mess" of points? Intuitively, it seems unreasonable. In reality, it is. It is merely a mathematical artifact to find that single best fitting line. Students accept the "solution" to the regression equation as the line you see in Figure 7–1B, but they have a hard time believing this line is the best representation of all those scattered points.

In fact, that straight line is often *not* the best representation of the data. A curved line (a nonlinear, or quadratic equation) might fit the data more

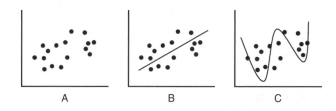

FIGURE 7–1 Fitting Linear (B) and Nonlinear (C) Equations to a Set of Data Points (A)

appropriately (see Figure 7–1C). Yet researchers are so anchored in a linear approach that it's often difficult to "think outside the line," and so, the solution is to look for interaction effects; however, the study of interaction effects in multiple regression is itself quite limited. Resnicow and Page (2008) sound the warning:

> In complex dynamic systems the interaction of factors can yield almost infinite potential patterns. In regression models, this degree of complexity may be analogous to higher-order interaction terms that could involve 5-, 10-, or 15-way interactions. Although linear methods can be used to model such interactions, they are limited statistically and conceptually. . . . Untangling a 3-way or higher-order interaction generally extends beyond our ability to map and interpret such a finding. . . . Linear models of behavior change may then be both conceptually inappropriate and statistically futile. (p. 1385–1386)

It is public health's (our) insistence in dealing with human behavior and behavior change from a linear perspective that might explain why the behavioral models we employ (and the research findings we encounter from testing these models) account for (or predict) so little of the variance in the behaviors examined. According to Resnicow and Page (2008), "The limitations of a rational-linear conceptualization of behavior change may . . . explain in part the modest proportion of behavioral variance accounted for in the literature (typically 10%–20% and rarely higher than 50%)" (p. 1382).

Why aren't nonlinear analyses then used more frequently than linear ones? I'm hard pressed to provide an accurate answer here because I really don't know, and I haven't seen studies focusing on this question (perhaps you could propose one?). My first guess would be the mathematical complexity of the models and perhaps the difficulty in interpreting some of the results. My second guess would be that health behavior scientists shy away from complexity and prefer straightforward, intuitive, and easily applicable answers to matters related to changing human behavior. If it is made too complex, then professionals/practitioners do not want to deal with it. Geez, we can't even handle quasi-complex statistical data analyses, at times, as researchers! We pray no one will propose even more complex ways of doing what we already find very difficult to do!

AN ALTERNATIVE

An alternative to such deliberate focus on human behavior as a linear process consists in adding nonlinear and complex systems ways of thinking about human health and illness to our theoretical repertoire (Gatrell, 2005). In fact, such a strategy dovetails nicely with the suggestions we made to counteract the exaggerated focus on individual-level factors.

Such a simple change—adding nonlinear approaches—may seem trivial; it may seem merely like adding another option to the smorgasbord of theories already before us, but it is not. For Resnicow and Page (2008), adopting a complex systems approach in public health "may require reconceptualizing how and why we influence change" (p. 1386). This approach leads, inevitably, to giving serious thought to health promotion's goals and strategies (or its means and ends). It also leads to important questions whether continuing to apply linear perspectives to complex realities is both ethical and safe, as Klaus Mainzer (1994) reminds us in his book *Thinking in Complexity: The Complex Dynamics of Matter, Mind, and Mankind*:

> Our approach suggests that physical, social, and mental reality is non-linear and complex. This essential result of synergetic epistemology demands severe consequences of our behavior. As we underlined, linear thinking may be dangerous in a nonlinear complex reality. . . . Our physicians and psychologists must learn to consider humans as complex non-linear entities of mind and body. Linear thinking may fail to yield a successful diagnosis. Local, isolated, and "linear" therapies of medical treatment may cause negative synergetic effects. In politics and history, we must remember that mono-causality may lead to dogmatism, intolerance, and fanaticism. As the ecological, economic, and political problems of mankind have become global, complex, and nonlinear, the traditional concept of individual responsibility is questionable. . . . In short: The complex system approach demands new consequences in *epistemology* and *ethics*. (p. 13)

Important beginnings—regarding epistemological and ethical changes—are emerging in both public health and several of the fields from which we normally borrow. Slowly, but consistently, public health, psychology, physiology, neuroscience, nursing, economics, sexuality education, and health care administration are beginning either to consider applying complex systems approaches to their research and practice or to reexamine existing research findings that suggest nonlinearity. Let's take a look at a few examples.

In a study of problem drinkers and the reasons they provided for drinking less when they were interviewed at a 1-year follow-up to treatment programs, Helen Matzger and her colleagues concluded the most frequently cited reasons behind the changes in drinking habits were completely nonlinear. Reasons people gave for drinking less were associated with random, unplanned elements, such as undergoing a traumatic experience or undergoing spiritual transformation. In the conclusion of their study, Matzger, Kaskutas, and Weisner (2005) wrote,

> For both the general population and treated samples [the study compared these groups], having experienced a negative/traumatic event (including hitting rock bottom) and having a spiritual awakening, each more than doubled an individual's odds of sustained remission from problem drinking. These results confirm findings from other studies that regardless of treatment, the road to recovery from alcohol problems is often initiated by a crisis or series of negative events. . . . In this study, as in one other, interventions by medical personnel and family members were either nonsignificant predictors or negatively related [more intervention, less success] to sustained improvement. . . . Treatment programs . . . geared towards fostering spiritual awakenings, for example, may have better success in achieving remission from problem drinking. (p. 1643, 1644)

Another study, conducted by Robert West and Taj Sohal (2006), tested the hypothesis whether the "prevailing model of smoking cessation (that smokers typically prepare their attempts to stop smoking in advance . . .) is correct" (West & Sohal, 2006, p. 458). Carried out in England, the study examined 918 smokers and 996 ex-smokers. An incisive test of the assumptions underlying the Stages of Change model (one of the most popular theoretical frameworks in public health, today; see Table 4–2 in Chapter 4), the findings indicated the model is *not* correct. In fact, West and Sohal (2006) argue:

> The results show that a substantial proportion of attempts to stop smoking are made without any previous planning and, surprisingly, that unplanned quit attempts have a greater chance of succeeding. . . .
>
> We hypothesize an alternative model to the stages of change approach, one that is based on "catastrophe theory." Catastrophe theory [one type of nonlinear theories] is a branch of mathematics that deals with the way in which tensions develop in systems so that even small triggers can lead to sudden "catastrophic" changes. We propose that beliefs, past experiences, and the current situation create varying levels of "motivational tension," in the presence of which even quite small "triggers" can lead to a renunciation of smoking. (p. 460)

Another example is this: In 2001, Byrne, Mazanov, and Gregson applied a nonlinear model to analyzing data for adolescent smoking behavior after teens participated in smoking-prevention programs. The sample included 1689 school-aged adolescents taking part in three different smoking-prevention programs in Australia. The authors ran statistical analyses comparing a series of linear regression models to another set of nonlinear equations. Although the linear models explained approximately 27% of the variance in smoking behavior among adolescents who took part in a prevention program, the nonlinear models were able to explain 45% of the variance (or of the changes) in their smoking practices. The authors conclude, after these comparisons, the nonlinear approach they used to model the data "provided a better fit for the data than did any of a number of simple or interactive linear models" (Byrne et al., 2001, p. 115). They also conclude:

> Overall, this study did not provide overwhelming support for the usefulness of smoking prevention programs in adolescence. While some program effects were statistically significant, the amount of variance modeled in smoking outcomes was not impressive, at least as revealed by linear models. (pp. 132–133)

This last quote highlights the potential benefits nonlinear analyses may bring to evaluating health promotion interventions: When most of our program evaluations find small effects (or little variance explained) resulting from the intervention, do these findings actually reflect the truth about the programs? Could it be, instead, that our evaluations—because they employ mostly linear statistics for analyses—simply do not "capture" the actual changes? The Australian study employed post-hoc analyses of data from three smoking prevention programs. The authors noted their study suffered from important limitations because the variables they used had been measured within a linear framework; in other words, the data were not intended for a nonlinear statistical analysis. Nevertheless, even with this important weakness, the analysis was able to demonstrate substantially more variability (change) in participants' smoking behavior than was originally detected with the linear regression models. Does this provide a clue that nonlinear approaches might be the best way to analyze program effectiveness? We need more tests of this hypothesis, for sure.

A REMINDER AND A REALITY CHECK

Having advocated for health promotion to shift to more complexity-science-focused theories, it is important that I end this section with a couple of cautionary notes, or reality checks (whatever you wish to call them). First, as

Resnicow and Page (2008) remind us, nonlinear approaches should not override linearity entirely:

> The linear and quantum paradigms are not necessarily mutually exclusive. Our view of behavior change can include both complex and chaotic processes as well as those that are more linear and rational. . . . Specifically, some behavior change events may best be explained as simple linear phenomena, whereas others may be highly complex and nonlinear. . . . Some individuals may, by their nature, be prone to employ linear or rational decision-making processes typically associated with left-hemispheric functioning. Others may be predisposed to complex or quantum processes in which change is more unpredictable, dramatic, and less planned. (p. 1386)

There is a strong need to add nonlinear approaches to health promotion—especially given the evidence of modest effectiveness of our intervention programs—yet linearity has its proper place in the plethora of stories told about human beings. (I remember reading somewhere that linear approaches are especially useful, for instance, if you or I were to undergo brain surgery. In this scenario, we might very much appreciate it if the surgeon has a planned, step A to step B approach to cutting into our bodies!).

If it is important to heed to the warning Resnicow and Page offer us, it is also valuable to conduct a "reality check": While the good news is that complexity science allows us to examine human phenomena in ways that capture their dynamics, interactions, and changes, the bad news is sobering: Complexity science is still "in its infancy" (Zimmerman, Lindberg, & Plsek, 1998). Scientists are still struggling with issues of measurement, analyses, and overall support for the theories. Brug (2006) reminds us of this:

> I agree that the scientific evidence for the prevailing [linear] health behavioral theories may be weak for many nutrition and physical activity behaviors. However, the direct empirical evidence for a chaotic nature of such behaviors or the quantum leap character of behavior change is absent. (p. 3)

Even if evidence supporting the effectiveness of nonlinear approaches is still in developmental stages, scholars from various disciplines and fields of knowledge have glimpsed their potential. What they have grasped has moved them to call on their professional colleagues to consider this new perspective seriously. Examples of scholars summoning the field to adopt dynamic systems strategies and viewpoints abound. They can be found in areas such as nursing (Holden, 2005), social work (Burgess, 2004), psychiatry (Miller, 2004), embryology (Goodman, 1997), sexuality education (Boyer, 1998), health care administration (Forbes-Thompson,

Leiker, & Bleich, 2007), and education, among others (Cooper & Geyer, 2008). Although these calls have been put forth for at least a decade, if not longer, only recently has health promotion joined the chorus of professional fields being enticed/stirred to add a nonlinear, quantum viewpoint to its practice and research (Baranowski, 2006; Brug, 2006; Green, 2006; Resnicow & Page, 2008; Resnicow & Vaughan, 2006).

In addition to the lack of (but emergent) evidence, it is equally important to bear in mind that complexity science comprises more than one theory (Zimmerman, Lindberg, & Plsek, 1998):

> The science encompasses more than one theoretical framework. Complexity science is highly interdisciplinary including biologists, anthropologists, economists, sociologists, management theorists and many others in a quest to answer some fundamental questions about living, adaptable, changeable systems. (p. 5)

Personally, I don't see having a set of theories (instead of a single theory) as a problem, but you may, given how we have become used to applying single frameworks to our health promotion interventions and research. More on this topic of single versus multiple theories is provided in Chapter 9. For now, it may be helpful to keep in mind the need for multilevel approaches to health behaviors and the parallel importance of interdisciplinary and multidisciplinary strategies for promoting health. Complexity science certainly opens wide the doors to these multiple levels and to such integration of various perspectives.

Despite these realities and slow goings, I strongly believe the contributions nonlinear theories and complexity science can bring to health promotion practice greatly outweigh any of its potentially negative elements and, with time, will captivate the minds of public health. I agree wholeheartedly with Larry Green, Reniscow, and Page and make their pleas my own:

> This, then, is the hope we harbor and the plea we seem to be making to systems scientists: Bring your theoretical and methodological tools for network analysis, knowledge transfer approaches, and systems organizing methods (including participatory research) to help us [in public health] get a handle on the multiplicity of influences at work in the real world of practice, so that the evidence from our study of interventions and programs can reflect that complex reality rather than mask it. (Green, 2006, p. 406)
>
> We hope to encourage public health practitioners and researchers to incorporate nonlinear concepts into the design and analysis of their interventions. This goal may require adjusting our expectations for how well we can predict and quantify the change process; this means embracing these concepts rather than wrestling with them. (Resnicow & Page, 2008, p. 1388)

SUGGESTIONS FOR PRACTICING THEORETICAL THINKING

1. Perform a brief search of the health promotion literature; see which studies you can find that employ a nonlinear perspective, or approach, to the study's design, data analysis, and interpretation. Ask yourself how these studies differ from the linear approaches you have been more accustomed to reading (you may start by reading some of the studies I mention/cite in this chapter and use these to begin "pulling the thread" of similar publications).

2. Debate with some of your colleagues the reasons why health promotion has been so reluctant to adopt a nonlinear, dynamic approach to health promotion.

3. Consider the curriculum/program under which you have been trained. Ask yourself how, within that curriculum, nonlinear perspectives could be more systematically incorporated. How would you design a public health training program emphasizing complexity sciences?

REFERENCES

Baranowski, T. (2006). Crisis and chaos in behavioral nutrition and physical activity. *International Journal of Behavioral Nutrition and Physical Activity, 3,* 27.

Blackman, T. (2000). Complexity theory. In G. Browning, A. Halcli, & F. Webster (Eds.), *Understanding Contemporary Society: Theories of the Present* (pp. 139–150). London: Sage Publications.

Boyer, M. R. P. (1998). Chaos, complexity, and constant change: implications for education and learning. *Journal of Sex Education and Therapy, 23*(1), 105–108.

Brug, J. (2006). Order is needed to promote linear or quantum changes in nutrition and physical activity behaviors: a reaction to "A chaotic view of behavior change" by Resnicow and Vaughan. *International Journal of Behavioral Nutrition and Physical Activity, 3,* 29–32.

Buhi, E., Goodson, P., & Neilands, T. (2007). Structural equation modeling: a primer for health behavior researchers. *American Journal of Health Behavior, 31*(1), 74–85.

Burgess, H. (2004). Redesigning the curriculum for social work education: complexity, conformity, chaos, creativity, collaboration. *Social Work Education, 23*(2), 163–183.

Byrne, D. G., Mazanov, J., & Gregson, R. A. M. (2001). A Cusp Catastrophe analysis of changes to adolescent smoking behaviour in response to smoking prevention programs. *Nonlinear Dynamics, Psychology, and Life Sciences, 5*(2), 115–137.

Cooper, H., & Geyer, R. (2008). Using "complexity" for improving educational research in health care. *Social Science & Medicine, 67,* 177–182.

Forbes-Thompson, S., Leiker, T., & Bleich, M. R. (2007). High-performing and low-performing nursing homes: a view from complexity science. *Health Care Management Review, 32*(4), 341–351.

Gatrell, A. C. (2005). Complexity theory and geographies of health: a critical assessment. *Social Science & Medicine, 60,* 2661–2671.

Gleick, J. (1987). *Chaos: Making a New Science* (11th Printing, 1988 ed.). New York: Viking.

Goodman, R. E. (1997). Understanding human sexuality—specifically homosexuality and the paraphilias—in terms of chaos theory and fetal development. *Medical Hypotheses, 48,* 237–243.

Green, L. W. (2006). Public health asks of systems science: to advance our evidence-based practice, can you help us get more practice-based evidence? *American Journal of Public Health, 96,* 406–409.

Holden, L. M. (2005). Complex adaptive systems: concept analysis. *Journal of Advanced Nursing, 52*(6), 651–657.

Lincoln, Y., & Guba, E. G. (1985). *Naturalistic Inquiry.* Newbury Park, CA: Sage Publications.

Mainzer, K. (1994). *Thinking in Complexity: The Complex Dynamics of Matter, Mind and Mankind.* New York: Springer-Verlag.

Matzger, H., Kaskutas, L. A., & Weisner, C. (2005). Reasons for drinking less and their relationship to sustained remission from problem drinking. *Addiction, 100,* 1637–1646.

Miller, W. R. (2004). The phenomenon of quantum change. *Journal of Clinical Psychology/In Session, 60,* 453–460.

Resnicow, K., & Page, S. E. (2008). Embracing chaos and complexity: a quantum change for public health. *American Journal of Public Health, 98*(8), 1382–1389.

Resnicow, K., & Vaughan, R. (2006). A chaotic view of behavior change: a quantum leap for health promotion. *International Journal of Behavioral Nutrition and Physical Activity, 3.*

West, R., & Sohal, T. (2006). "Catastrophic" pathways to smoking cessation: findings from national survey. *British Medical Journal, 332,* 458–460.

Zimmerman, B. J. (2000a). *Comparing complexity science with traditional science,* 2008. Available from http://plexusinstitute.com/edgeware/archive/think/main_prim1.html

Zimmerman, B. J., Lindberg, C., Plsek, P. (1998). Edgeware: Insights from Complexity Science for Health Care Leaders. Irving: VHA Inc.

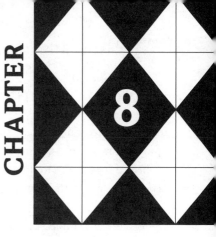

Applying Theory to Health Promotion Research

A WORD ABOUT GUIDELINES

We completed our journey through the current theoretical landscape in health promotion. I hope you found the trip interesting, at least. Ideally, you will have collected suggestions for how *you* could make a contribution to health promotion by filling in the theoretical gaps, the many "blind spots" encountered along the way.

Realistically, I hope the journey also prepared you to accept the fact that this theoretical landscape is what it is and that you and I have to deal with it, despite its imperfections. As much as we hope health promotion is becoming more influenced by systems-level theories, more balanced about its fixation on rationality, and less drawn to linear ways of thinking about human phenomena, the stark reality is what we have in front of us: The theories you saw listed in Chapter 4 are the most commonly used theories in the field today. Especially if you are a budding professional or a graduate student, at this point, it may be in your best interest to embrace what is familiar to your colleagues, show them you know how to think theoretically *within* familiar parameters, gain their respect and, after establishing yourself professionally, *then* instigate new lines of thinking, new theories, new ways of telling the stories about health, illness, and disease.

For now, however, let's consider some very pragmatic questions, of vital importance: *How does one apply theory to research or to the development and evaluation of health promotion programs? How does one "use" these health promotion theories that the textbooks describe? How does one even* choose *a theory, or theories, to be used?* To respond to these questions, I would like to offer you some guidelines.

When I perform a quick examination of the term "guideline" in *Roget's Thesaurus of English Words and Phrases"* (MICRA Inc., 1991), I find 41 different dimensions to its meaning! Among these are the ideas of direction, journey, advice, information, straightness, limit, method, and measurement. Based on these various dimensions of meaning, I would like to propose that the guidelines I will offer you in this chapter are *not* rules set in stone, procedures to be followed in a lock-step fashion. They are merely suggestions of direction, of paths to take in your journey into the world of theory—simply a bit of advice and information that might help you set limits and find your way through theory-grounded research and practice. That's all. Keep in mind that these steps are not rigid. Actually, quite the opposite: They are iterative and synergistic. You'll find yourself going back and forth across some of the guidelines; you will also have the experience that completing one step may intensify (or amplify) the effects of a previous step; when/if you return to earlier steps, to repeat or add to them, they will already look a bit different than they did the first time, making that step a bit easier the second time around.

Furthermore, (1) don't expect these guidelines to cover every single contingency, every circumstance you may face in your research, and (2) don't lock yourself into these guidelines: Explore ways to make them work for you, for your projects; adapt them, and create your own professional "*modus operandi.*" After you've developed and established your own pathways, discard these guidelines.

Each set of guidelines I propose in this chapter can be found in an abbreviated, checklist format at the end of the chapter; so you can actually "check off" each of the steps as you complete them. Also, in this chapter, I cover the *application of theory to research* exclusively. Applying theory to program planning and evaluation will be covered in the next chapter. I also should warn you about how I numbered the sections in this chapter. To facilitate your navigation and to help you figure out which set of guidelines you're dealing with, I chose to break the rules for outlining sections in chapters using letters and numbers (such as *A.1*, and *A.1.a*). Instead, I chose to number the headings devoted to quantitative research with the initials QT; the ones in the qualitative section, with QL, and the mixed-methods portion, with MM.

Finally, keep in mind that the guidelines provided in this chapter (and the next) are intended to serve as *tools* when you actively engage in conducting your own research. You may, for this reason, choose not to read the entire chapter but instead focus on the sections that seem more relevant to *your* project. If, however, you are not engaged in research at this moment but wish to understand how theory is used in different types of research, by all means, you're welcome to read the entire chapter! I hope you find it useful, yes, but *more than useful.* My wish is that you actually learn something more about theory and come to admit, "I never thought about it *that* way!" (Sometimes I think I've become addicted to hearing my students say this!)

APPLYING THEORY TO RESEARCH—AN OVERVIEW

Students in my Theories of Health Behavior class have no trouble understanding the stories being told by most health promotion theories. The students do a fine job regurgitating all of the constructs for a given theory, for instance, the Transtheoretical Model, in a written exam. They also do well when comparing theories and identifying each one's strengths, weaknesses, and potential. Yet nearly all of these students have a difficult time deciding which theories to employ when conducting their own research after the class is over. For some reason—and I do concede the reason may be that I haven't been able to teach this clearly—students struggle with choosing the most appropriate theory for their research project or for the program they plan to implement. Apparently, I'm not the only one witnessing this struggle: Noel Brewer and Barbara Rimer also refer to this in one of the chapters they authored for the Glanz book (Brewer & Rimer, 2008):

> This complexity [involved in choosing theories] has prompted students as close as Chapel Hill, North Carolina, and as far as Iran and China to pose versions of the same question to us about theory: *"How do you pick one theory over another?"* (p. 151)

One of the reasons students worldwide struggle with choosing theories might be that theory application is, in fact, quite a difficult task and especially difficult to perform *appropriately*, given that in the world of theory, the notions of "right" or "wrong" don't apply; only the ideas of "adequate" or " inadequate"; "useful" or "useless." It might be because of its difficulty that it is rare to see the process of choosing or applying theory to health promotion research and practice described in sufficient detail.

In fact, when we closely examine the theory textbooks I described in Chapter 4, we find that most of them write in very general terms about applying theory to research and practice. When it comes to offering specific strategies, guidelines, or step-by-step procedures, only Joanna Hayden's (2009) book *Introduction to Health Behavior Theory* contains an entire chapter dedicated to "Choosing a Theory" (Chapter 10). Granted, Edberg's (2007) book *Social and Behavioral Theory in Public Health* guides readers to think about application throughout the entire book, but he does it by discussing a specific theory, asking questions about how it relates to theory or practice, and offering the application "solution" as it relates to *that* theory (or theories) discussed in *that* chapter.

Most theory texts in health promotion do little to actually help readers *choose and use* a theory. More has been written about applying theory to practice—because for this type of application, we have very useful tools such as the PRECEDE–PROCEED model or Intervention Mapping—but little is available on how to choose theory for research, how to derive hypotheses from the theory, and how to use the theory to assist with data analysis (primary or secondary data).

Because Joanna Hayden (2009) does indeed provide a set of guidelines (my hat's off to her for offering these to her readers!), let's examine them. She introduces the chapter on choosing a theory by saying this:

> Knowing some of the many different theories and models that can be used to explain health behavior is one thing—knowing which theory to use when is another. Unfortunately, there is no magic formula or chart to tell you which of the theories is just right for a given situation, because there are no right or wrong theories. (p. 135)

To facilitate this complex task of choosing which theory is more appropriate for a given "situation," she provides the following guidelines (and a chart) to help readers narrow their choices (Hayden, 2009, p. 135):

1. Identify the health issue or problem and the population affected.
2. Gather information about the issue or population or both.
3. Identify possible reasons or causes for the problem.
4. Identify the level of interaction (intrapersonal, interpersonal, or community) under which the reasons or causes most logically fit.
5. Identify the theory or theories that best match the level and the reasons or causes.

While these steps may seem intuitive and feasible, I would argue they are problematic because Hayden suggests readers "identify possible reasons or causes for the problem" (guideline 3), when such identification is the job, or the role, of the *theory itself*, not yours. Hayden's guidelines, as I see them, function like this: I give you a recipe for making chocolate chip cookies, and one of the steps in the recipe is to get a bag of chocolate chip cookies, break them into small pieces, and mix them into the dough. If you were following the recipe you would certainly (at least I hope you would!) stop and say, "Huh? If I'm making chocolate chip cookies, it means I don't have any chocolate chip cookies. If I had any, I wouldn't be making them!" Hayden's guidelines for applying theory do the same as my chocolate chip cookie recipe: They ask that *you do something*—identify possible reasons or causes for the problem—that constitutes precisely what the *theory should do for you*; theories identify possible reasons or causes. They tell stories about the factors that influence or affect certain phenomena. Your job is to find the theory making most sense for your problem/phenomenon of interest and see whether the theory identifies (*for you*) the "possible reasons or causes for the problem." So, as glad as I was to see *someone* talking about strategies for choosing appropriate theories, I felt disappointed that Hayden's guidelines make us rely on store-bought cookies.

I do want to offer, therefore, some guidelines of my own: Guidelines for *choosing* and *applying* theory to research and to practice. I will attempt to be as practical and "user friendly" as possible, but I must warn you that it takes work. Well, anything worth doing takes a lot of work, as you should well know by now. You wouldn't be reading this book if you didn't believe the same thing!

Before I present my set of guidelines for choosing and applying a theory to your research project, however, I must first ask the question: "*What approach are you taking in your research?*" By approach, I mean what *kind* of research will you be doing? To which paradigm will your inquiry belong: quantitative (also referred to as *positivistic*), qualitative (also known as *naturalistic*), or a mixed methods (also called *pragmatist*) approach (Onwuegbuzie & Leech, 2005a, 2005b)? You may react by thinking, "But these approaches apply only to the *methods* I'll be using in my study, not to the theory . . . only to how I will collect data, and to what type of data I will be collecting and analyzing. For theory, it doesn't matter whether I'm collecting quantitative data (in the form of numbers), or qualitative data (in the form of text, or words)."

Well, all I can say is this: "You wish!" Unfortunately, reality is more complex than we anticipate: Theory plays very different roles in the different research paradigms (as we see in the next sections). It *behaves* differently, and you will *use it* differently in each of them. That's why the question is important. Do you know the answer regarding the research project you have in mind? If so, here we go: I'll discuss the role and then the guidelines for choosing and applying theory in each of the three research paradigms. If you don't know the answer to the approach or paradigm question, I recommend you discuss this with a mentor/colleague, or take additional research methods courses to learn more about these different approaches.

THE ALTERNATIVE: A-THEORETICAL RESEARCH

Regardless of which approach you choose (quantitative, qualitative, or mixed methods), keep in mind the alternative: a-theoretical research. Mark Dressman (2008), in his book *Using Social Theory in Educational Research*, invites us to consider the advantages in using theory as a roadmap:

> A great advantage of having a well-developed theoretical framework before one begins analyzing data and writing up a research project is the direction and focus theory can give to these processes. To understand how this is so, imagine the collection and analysis of data for a study without an explicit theoretical perspective. (p. 116)

Dressman proceeds by describing a simple example of educational research. I will follow his lead by offering you a simple example of health promotion research: Say you wished to research the topic of childhood obesity, but you were specifically interested in the mechanisms through which the parents' obesity might influence their child's weight gain. What information would you need to obtain in order to answer your questions about parental factors influencing childhood obesity? What data would you collect? Where would you even begin to collect data: at the families' doctors' office from their medical charts? At the children's schools? At family gatherings? At home during meal times? What data would you gather: parents' perceptions of how they might influence their children's obesity? Children's reasoning for their food choices? School teachers' views of the dynamics within each child's family? As Dressman (2008) highlights, without a theoretical framework, we feel tempted to collect data on everything, without even knowing what "everything" might be:

> And, once "everything" had been collected, where and how would the analysis begin? How would a researcher begin to organize the data, to know what likely patterns to look for, and to recognize patterns that were unlikely? What would determine what was considered "likely" or "unlikely"? What would constitute a pattern? (p. 115)

You get the point: Without theory, a researcher engages in a mapless journey—an arduous, long, and (at times) exhausting trip without any direction or sign posts to ensure that he/she reaches the destination through the most efficient route. Therefore, as we struggle with the complex task of ensuring our research projects and our intervention programs are theory-based, we must remind ourselves we do this for one very simple reason: so our research and our program planning make sense and have purpose, while saving us a lot of time and grief in the process.

QT—APPLYING THEORY TO QUANTITATIVE (OR POSITIVISTIC) RESEARCH

Because the scope of this book doesn't allow me to present a detailed, in-depth background to quantitative (or positivistic) research, I will only highlight some of its major characteristics so you may better understand the role that theory plays within this research paradigm.

Although most of us think of positivism as a way of doing science, positivism also refers to a collection of philosophical ideas, or a philosophical movement. This movement, in the early 19th century, was perceived as having the "potential for the reform of such diverse areas as ethics, religion, and politics, in addition to philosophy" (Lincoln & Guba, 1985, p. 19). The strongest impact the movement eventually had, however, was neither on philosophy, ethics, or politics; positivism's strongest impact was felt in *science*. Lincoln and Guba (1985) explain, "The concepts of positivism provided a new rationale for the doing of science that amounted to a literal paradigm revolution" (p. 19).

What—you may be asking—were these ideas, powerful enough to promote such a revolution? In their book *Naturalistic Inquiry*, Yvonna Lincoln and Egon Guba (1985) outline five major basic beliefs held by positivists, which deeply influenced the *doing* of science, in modern times:

1. Beliefs regarding the nature of reality (ontology)—There is a single tangible reality "out there" fragmentable into independent variables and processes, any of which can be studied independently of the others; inquiry can converge onto that reality until, finally, it [the reality] can be predicted and controlled.

2. Beliefs regarding the relationship of knower to known (epistemology)—The inquirer and the object of inquiry are independent; the knower and the known constitute a discrete dualism.

3. Beliefs regarding the possibility of generalization—The aim of inquiry is to develop a nomothetic [law-like] body of knowledge in the form of generalizations that are truth statements free from both time and context (they will hold anywhere and at any time).

4. Beliefs regarding the possibility of causal linkages—Every action can be explained as the result (effect) of a real cause that precedes the effect temporally (or is at least simultaneous with it).

5. Beliefs regarding the role of values in inquiry (axiology)—Inquiry is value-free and can be guaranteed to be so by virtue of the objective methodology employed. (pp. 36–38)

QT1—The Role of Theory in Quantitative (Positivistic) Research

Given this set of axioms, or basic beliefs, it is not difficult to conclude that the role of theory within a positivist approach consists in providing explanations that, ultimately, allow prediction and control of the researched phenomena; these explanations are developed "objectively" by value-neutral theorists/researchers and explain cause-and-effect relationships that can be generalized to any phenomenon, regardless of its context. The ultimate goal is to turn these explanations, as much as possible, into universal "laws."

Positivistic or quantitative research usually (but not always) *begins* with theory. After identifying a problem, issue, or question requiring attention, the first step is to search for theories that might explain what the researcher observes. The first significant moment in a research design, therefore, involves active listening: What are others saying about this issue/problem? What's the nature of the conversation other scholars are having, about this topic? Which explanations or solutions are these scholars proposing? Thus, an inventory of the ongoing conversation about the topic of interest is—from a positivistic or quantitative research perspective— the essential first step. Skipping this step, or choosing to ignore the conversation being exchanged around them, is a big mistake many researchers make. A mistake akin to deciding to purchase a new car without doing one's "homework," without collecting any information about it, without reading any consumers' reviews about specific models. Not recommended, say the quantitative researchers in the field.

But how *does* one do one's homework, and how *does* one use theory in quantitative research? Later here, you will find my set of guidelines for choosing a theory, for grounding your research question(s) or hypotheses in that theory, and for applying theory to the analyses of your data.

QT2—Choosing a Theory (or Theories) for Your Quantitative Research Project

Here are the steps to follow, in order to choose the theory (or theories) you may want to use.

Guidelines and Tips: Choosing a Theory for Your Quantitative Research Project

1. Name the problem or the issue that you wish to explore or examine in your research project.
2. Conduct a cursory search of the scientific literature related to your problem/issue/phenomenon. Author John Creswell (1988) recommends your search be discipline specific:

> If the unit of analysis for variables is individuals, look in the psychology literature; to study groups or organizations, look in the sociological literature. If the project examines individuals and groups, consider the social psychology literature. Of course, other discipline theories may be useful (e.g., to study an economic issue, the theory may be found in economics). (p. 90)

TIP

Search for published reviews of the topic. To do this, add the words "review" or "systematic review" or "meta-analysis" to your search terms. Choose the most recently published reviews. Read these, first.

3. After you searched for reviews and also found several research reports related to the problem/issue you wish to study, read the articles you identified.

TIP

Read the articles in chronological order, from oldest to most recently published. This allows you to observe the "progression" or the development of the topic over time.

4. As you read each article, make a note of which theoretical framework each study employed.

TIP

Develop a table (or matrix) to capture information for each article you read (Garrard, 2004). Table 8–1 gives you an example of a table you can use to capture the information about theory (or any other data you wish to extract from each report you read). (I develop my matrices in MS Word, but some people prefer other software.)

5. In the matrix you developed, also make note of the constructs and variables being examined in each study you read.
6. Examine your matrix after you have read between 5 and 10 published reports, and consider the theories being used, as well as the variables/constructs being explored.
7. Begin identifying potential "candidate theories."

TIP

Ask yourself—as you read and complete your matrix:

a. Do any of the theories being used in these studies appear applicable to *my* research question, to my research project?
b. Do any of the studies I read examine constructs or variables that are very similar to what I would like to examine in my own research?
c. Is there a *pattern* to the theories being used? In other words, does one theory tend to be used more frequently than others, or are the theories "all over the place"?

Table 8–1 Sample Matrix for Collecting Information Regarding Individual Studies' Use of Theory

Authors	Year	Title	Citation	Variables Studied	Theories Employed	Note to Self	Location
Smith, J., & Jones, B.	2008	Factors influencing young adults' adherence to moderate exercise recommendations.	*Journal of Exercise and Diet*, Vol. 9(3), 1–15	Self-efficacy Intention Attitudes Subjective Norms	Theory of Planned Behavior Self-Efficacy Theory	Authors' use of theory is rather straightforward. They do a good job of presenting a brief description of both theories, and defining all of the constructs.	I have a pdf copy of this article at: H:\Literature\ Young adults' adherence to exercise .pdf
Cary, R., & Dressler, T.	2007	What works to promote exercise among young adults?	*Exercise Mentality*, Vol. 20(4), 24–28.	Perceptions of seriousness of not exercising/consequences Perceptions of confidence in exercising regularly	Health Belief Model Self Efficacy Theory	This article's use of theory is not as clearcut as in the previous one. The theories are not named, but one citation points to the HBM. Self-efficacy theory is not mentioned by name, but the construct of self-efficacy is clearly defined, with a citation to the theory's main text by A. Bandura.	I have a pdf copy of this article at: H:\Literature\ Motivation to exercise .pdf

8. After you've identified a couple of possible "candidate theories," search the reference section of the articles you've read and see whether the authors cited original sources for those theories.

TIP

Oftentimes, the full exposition of a theory will happen in a *book*, instead of a journal article, so pay close attention to the citations. Consult the referenced books whenever you can: Usually, they will have the complete development of the theory, with detailed definitions and explanations of the constructs and their theoretical relationships.

9. After identifying one or two candidate theories, spend some time reading and learning about them.

TIP

Don't merely *read* about a theory; *write* your thoughts, reactions, and gut feelings about it *as you read*. You can use your matrix to capture your thoughts for each theory if you'd like (notice the "Notes to Self" column in the matrix in Table 8-1). This way, your matrix will store all the information pertaining to each study and each theory, along with your thoughts, reactions, and questions.

10. Select the theory/theories you will employ in your study.

Troubleshooting
What if after you follow the steps I outlined (1) you have too many potential candidate theories or (2) you don't have enough potential candidates or the published research is quite "a-theoretical"? What then? Let's tackle one problem at a time.

Too Many Theories
First, if you have too many interesting theories, all of them appearing as suitable candidates to ground your research project, asking yourself these questions may help you decide the following:

1. Which theory do I understand better? Which one "clicks" with my way of thinking? Which one makes most sense to me? Which tells the most interesting story?
2. With which theory is the field more comfortable? Which one will be easiest to explain to my colleagues when I try to publish my study's report? Which one will be more acceptable in the ongoing professional conversation about this topic?

3. Which theory does my advisor, committee chair, principal investigator in a project, or other people exercising authority over my work know best? Which theory are people in my dissertation committee or in my research team more familiar with? Remember that having available expertise is an important resource to consider. You may want to break new ground and "push the envelope" in your theoretical perspective, but if you don't have expert backup, you may find yourself quite alone when trying to make sense of your data using the theory you chose.

Using Multiple Theories

A common practice in public health research is the use of multiple theories in a single research project. Researchers often employ various theories because each one appears to explain "portions" of the phenomena. At times, more than one theory is employed because the researcher wishes to explain the phenomenon from multiple levels (using an ecological approach) and requires, therefore, a mix of, for instance, individual-level and organization-level theories.

Is this "smorgasbord" approach to theories appropriate? Should we continue the practice that has become so common in our field? These are questions my students often bring to me, with much concern. And the answer is—as with most of these kinds of questions—far from clear cut: If it were not an acceptable practice, we probably would not see such a large number of studies that employ this approach published in reputable journals in our field.

On the other hand, this "collage" approach tends to turn the theorists who developed them on their graves (if they are dead) and to seriously aggravate those who are still alive. Why? Because using a few constructs of one theory, combined with a few other constructs selected from another theory, does little to test any particular theory fully; therefore, it defeats one of the main purposes of quantitative/positivist science: that of testing a theory and striving to make it more and more "universal" or generalizable.

The answer, therefore, to the question of whether it is appropriate to develop conceptual models (and hypotheses) based on various theories is this: *It depends.* It depends on whom you ask: If you ask public health scholars, concerned mainly with solving problems, designing interventions, and evaluating these interventions' effectiveness, they will tell you there's really no problem. What matters is that the approach *works:* It works to explain the phenomenon. It works to provide specific targets for intervention. It works to solve the problem at hand. Not much else besides this pragmatic approach matters: even if the theories chosen contradict each other regarding philosophical perspectives, basic beliefs, or essential values. If it works, it works.

If, however, you ask theorists themselves, or scholars concerned about going beyond immediate problem solving to enhancing the knowledge-base in the field, the answer to the question of appropriateness in using multiple theories might be quite different. These scholars might point out that the strongest contribution a research project can make is to provide empirical tests of a theory as a whole or to provide more evidence of how a specific theory—in its entirety—"behaves" within various contexts.

Yet, even if we consider these very different approaches to the application of multiple theories to public health research, we must concede this point: In order to conduct multilevel or ecological-based research in health promotion, there is no way but to invoke more than one theory. One could say: "But the theories being chosen for an ecological-based research project can remain intact at each of the levels they are being applied!" Yes, that is true: Let's say, for example, a researcher chooses to examine the problem of managing type I diabetes among children in socioeconomic minority groups employing an ecological, multilevel approach. This researcher might choose the Health Belief Model to explain the intrapersonal factors related to the children's perceptions of their diabetes and to explain the intrapersonal factors related to the parents' perceptions of their children's diabetes. The researcher may also examine the children's school policies regarding management of chronic conditions during the school hours; he or she may also select a community-focused theory to help understand the availability of appropriate health care for these children. And so on. . . .

In the previous example, despite having chosen at least three different types of theories, the researcher still must entertain the question of whether he or she will be using the theory as a whole (at each level) or will chop up the theories and focus only on select factors from each one. Granted, this latter option always seems more palatable; if nothing else, because the sheer number of factors involved (when one uses the theories "intact") becomes a deterrent for the researcher in terms of the *amount of data*, he or she will need to collect, analyze, and interpret.

The take-home point is this: One of the main contributions positivistic quantitative research can make to the existing body of knowledge in a given field is to provide tests of a particular theory. In contrast to what happens in health promotion practice, in research, theories should be—as much as possible—used as a whole. Here is what Hochbaum, Sorensen, and Lorig (1992) have to say about this:

> Theories are not simple lists of variables each of which by itself somehow determines an outcome. Theories deal with the interaction of variables, and

it is this interaction of *all the theory's variables* that are supposed to bring predicted results. We have seen . . . that, for instance, according to the theory, neither self-efficacy nor value expectancy by itself can be expected to result in some desired outcome: both conditions need to be satisfied. *The most effective utilization of a theory, therefore, would entail its application in toto.* (p. 309)

Not Enough Theories

If, however, during your review of the literature you encounter little or close to nothing in terms of theoretical frameworks being applied to your topic of interest (and this will be the case more frequently than I care to admit), then things get a bit more complex. I propose these suggestions for troubleshooting this problem:

1. Examine the theories with which you are most familiar (theories you learned about in your courses; theories your colleagues are using; theories you've read about in readings not related to your project).
2. Consider whether any of these theories might help explain what you wish to examine/explore.
3. Examine the research in other fields; see whether anyone is doing anything remotely similar to what you're doing. For instance, if you wish to explore the role of emotions on decision making regarding risky choices, you will find quite a bit of theory being proposed in the field of economics or consumer behavior studies; not as many in health promotion or public health.

Keep in mind, however: when public health lacks solid theoretical frameworks to explain a phenomenon of interest, this is when you have the opportunity to innovate and make a theoretical contribution to the field. Explore outside-the-box alternatives. Such exploring usually means more work for you, yes, but makes your contribution more valuable in the short and long terms.

QT3—Grounding Your Research Questions and Hypotheses

After you have identified the theory that most appropriately explains or appears to best capture the phenomenon you wish to research, what do you do? How do you apply the theory to your research plan/proposal and, later to the reporting of your findings? First, let's consider a few steps that you can take to connect the theory you chose to your research questions or hypotheses.

**Guidelines and Tips: Grounding Your Research Questions
and Hypotheses**

1. Begin writing. Write a couple of paragraphs *naming* and *briefly describing* the theory you have chosen.

Provide . . .

a. The "official" and complete name of the theory (not the name by which it might be known in the field; those are often nicknames we give to our favorite models/frameworks)

b. The names of its main proponents (the scholars who developed the theory)

c. Dates for when the original/seminal work was published

d. Citations for some of the classic, *original* work (avoid citing textbooks, such as the Glanz book if you can; these books often present summaries of the theories written by authors other than the original theorists)

e. A brief description of what the theory addresses (e.g., "This theory addresses three factors influencing people's intention to behave in healthy/unhealthy ways: attitudes, perceived subjective norms, and perceived behavioral control; the theory hypothesizes "intention" as the strongest predictor of health behavior.")

2. Continue writing: write one paragraph identifying the theory's *main assumptions* and another paragraph presenting *your assumptions about the research topic*. According to Shoemaker, Tankard, and Lasorsa (2004), assumptions are theoretical statements that researchers take for granted. Assumptions sometimes cannot be tested scientifically, so they are accepted as unquestioned "truths." These are the "preconceptions" (some would say, "prejudices") we bring to our studies as researchers. Shoemaker et al. (2004) remind us

> It is helpful for scholars to clarify their own deeply held beliefs and to acknowledge these when directly pertinent to the study. The more scholars can identify the assumptions that underlie their theories and research, the more they and others can understand the implications of the theories. If the reader does not agree with the basic assumptions underlying the research, then the rest of the work is called into question. (p. 39)

Unfortunately, as Shoemaker and her co-authors highlight, identifying assumptions and describing them are perhaps the most difficult tasks related to applying theory. It's akin to asking fish to describe their liquid habitats; they see *through* the water and therefore are unable to see the water itself (Shoemaker et al., 2004):

> Identifying and stating assumptions is one of the most difficult parts of theory building because the things we take for granted are part of our individual ideological and normative systems and are therefore transparent to our daily thought processes. Such preconscious ideas have a direct effect on the research conducted. (p. 39)

Examples of assumptions underlying the research we conduct in health promotion include: health is a human right; economic development fosters better overall health for population groups; human beings can change their unhealthy behaviors into healthy ones if they choose to do so; factors once viewed as "character flaws"—such as excessive drinking, gambling, violent behavior—are now understood to be health-related conditions and/or medical problems.

TIP

To help identify and describe the assumptions made by your theory, and the ones *you* might hold, ask yourself these questions:

a. What are the basic beliefs this theory is built upon?

b. What are *my* basic beliefs about the topic I'm researching? What are my natural biases, the preconceived notions I bring to this study, the prejudices (positive or negative) I hold regarding this topic?

3. Continue writing: identify, define, and explain each of the factors you wish to examine in your study.

TIP

When you write, provide for your reader . . .

a. A conceptual definition (or, as I like to refer to it, a "dictionary-definition") of each construct, or factor, you will be examining. You should be able to find this definition in the theory itself.

b. An operational definition, or how *you* will measure that variable in your study. Shoemaker et al. (2004) explain operational definition as the "complete and explicit information about how the concept will be measured. This term can be confusing, because the word *definition* doesn't bring *measurement* to mind" (p. 29).

4. Continue writing: provide your study's theoretical statements (Shoemaker et al., 2004). In other words, describe relationships among the factors you chose to examine.

> **TIP**
>
> Provide readers with . . .
>
> a. A brief notion of how the theory explains the relationships among constructs (e.g., intention is the strongest predictor of behavior—how does the Theory of Planned Behavior *explain* this relationship between intention and behavior?).
>
> b. An explanation of what that relationship might look like in your particular study (e.g., "In this study, intention to exercise for 20 minutes, 3 times a week, will be the strongest predictor of this sample's adherence to a new exercise program"). In other words, avoid only "talking theory"; provide examples. These examples should come from your own research. This is how you begin to "tie" the theory to your study or to "ground" your research in the theory you chose.

5. Next, write down your study's main research question and/or hypotheses. You wish to provide the reader with at least one paragraph that very "tightly" focuses on the bottom-line research question you wish to answer. Because most research projects often have more than one question they try to address, you may wish to present your project as one question plus several related hypotheses—in other words, one take-home sound bite (to borrow from telecommunications language) and a couple of probes.

6. When writing hypotheses, focus on describing relationships among the *values* of your variables (think "quantity" here). Remember hypotheses are "guesstimates" you make about the quantified relationships that will emerge among factors in *your* particular study.

> **TIP**
>
> You may describe these relationships by writing about . . .
>
> a. *Expected differences* between the values of each of the variables (e.g., people in the treatment group—receiving the educational intervention—will *score higher* on the Quality of Life scale than people in the control group).
>
> b. *Expected effects* of one variable, on the other variable. For example, if attitudes toward genetic testing in the U.S. population change, the demand for genetic services may also change.

You can find very good treatments of how to word research questions and hypotheses in most research methods textbooks. I also highly recommend Shoemaker, Tankard, and Lasorsa's book *How to Build Social Science Theories* for more details on distinguishing between assumptions, theoretical propositions, and hypotheses. If you follow the previous guidelines and write a paragraph or two as I recommended, you will have accomplished quite a lot in terms of linking your research topic to the theory you chose. You will have demonstrated your ability to think theoretically about your topic, your ability to connect the chosen theory to the constructs or variables you wish to measure, and your skill in identifying assumptions laying hidden both in the theory and in your own belief-system. If you do these things, I promise you: your readers (including thesis/dissertation committee members) will be duly impressed.

QT4—Applying Theory to Data Analysis in Quantitative (Positivistic) Research

Even after graduate students (and many senior researchers) do a good job of grounding their research questions/hypotheses in the theory they chose, that theory mysteriously disappears from the project when the procedures and the results are described. Sometimes, if we're lucky, the theory is resurrected in the final portions of the research report in the discussion section. But we often have better luck at winning the lottery; very frequently, once the theory has been proposed as part of the introduction and background to the study, it is conveniently retired and forgotten. Yet, theory maintains its role as a roadmap, a tour guide if you will, throughout the entire quantitative research project. It is *especially* during the data analysis phase that it can be most helpful to the researcher. Unfortunately, our training programs have not done a very good job of teaching how to apply theory to data analysis.

The guidelines I propose in this section were developed by another faculty member who found herself quite disillusioned by her students' inability to connect theory and analysis. The solution to her disappointment was to write a book: *Theory-Based Data Analysis for the Social Sciences*. In it, the author—Carol Aneshensel (2002)—points to the nearly virtual absence of technical help for connecting social science theory to data analyses in research projects. She describes this dilemma in the preface:

> [After examining a student's preliminary doctoral exam] I was struck, not for the first time, by a technically correct description of a series of statistical techniques that had little relevance to the theory to be tested in the proposed research. Lest students think they have been unfairly singled out, I should mention that this disconnection is also found in the proposals of more seasoned investigators. I was puzzled because the students who struggled most with their data analysis were uniformly bright, articulate in their understanding of theory, and, most perplexingly, well trained in the techniques of multivariate statistics. This pattern

suggested that something was missing from the way we were training the next generation of social scientists. (p. xvii)

It would make little sense for me to describe Aneshensel's book in its entirety here; therefore, I'm going to merely summarize some of her suggestions, hoping these will open the doors for you to investigate, with more depth, how to move beyond statistical data analysis and, in fact, connect your study's data to your theory. Some of Aneshensel's recommendations for connecting theory to data analysis in quantitative (positivistic) research are outlined later here.

Guidelines and Tips: Applying Theory to Data Analysis in Quantitative (Positivistic) Research

I have borrowed the wording of these guidelines (presented as italicized text) and many of the ideas I share here with you directly from Carol Aneshensel's book:

1. *Assess whether the focal independent variable is associated with the dependent variable in the manner predicted by theory and at a level beyond chance* (Aneshensel, 2002, p. 235). Carol Aneshensel defines the "focal relationship" proposed by a theory as "the one relationship of primary significance—the heart of the theory" (p. 11). The focal relationship represents the association between the focal dependent and independent variables (DV/IV) in a study. Even multivariate studies will have an underlying focal relationship to be explored; sometimes that relationship is between a *set* of independent variables, and a *set* of dependent variables, but even then, there is one association that demands the researcher's focus, as the primary relationship to be tested. Statistically, there are many ways to test whether an association exists, and to determine whether the relationship is direct or mediated (Baron & Kenny, 1986).

   Statistically testing whether the focal relationship is merely a chance occurrence or has a strong probability of happening because there truly is a relationship helps you begin to assess your theory. When you find the relationship has a stronger-than-change probability of occurring, according to Aneshensel (2002),

   > This step establishes the feasibility of the focal relationship by showing that the values on the dependent variable correspond to the values on the independent variable in the *manner anticipated by the theory* and in a manner that is not likely to be just a chance occurrence. If not, our theory is discredited and should be critically revisited before proceeding with any analysis. (p. 236, emphasis mine)

The idea is not to "fish around" the data, searching for potential relationships that might be statistically significant: Start with the relationship the theory proposed. If possible, begin with only the two main variables and estimate (for instance, through regression analysis) the "bivariate association between the focal independent and dependent variables" (Aneshensel, 2002, p. 235). Test whether the probability of that relationship happening, is stronger than chance.

2. *Eliminate alternative explanations for the observed associations through the use of control and other independent variables* (Aneshensel, 2002, p. 235). This addresses the "third variable" problem, or in other words, it clarifies whether the relationship between variables A and B is not, in fact, explained or affected by the existence of variable C. For instance, I may have proposed, as the focal relationship in my study, that parents' attitudes toward sexuality directly affect their teenagers' sexual behavior(s). Yet, in my model, I also have the construct "perceived peer sexual behaviors" (or perceptions of what the teenager's friends do). There is a strong possibility that parents' attitudes have somewhat of a weaker effect on their teenagers' sexual behavior than we expect because what seems to really count are the perceptions that teenagers have of what their friends are doing, sexually speaking. "Perceived peer sexual behaviors" may then behave as a "third variable" in my study, attenuating or "toning down" the relationship between my originally proposed focal variables.

TIP

Add other variables (control or independent variables) to the regression equation that you used to test the focal relationship. Look for this:

a. What happened to the coefficient of that first focal independent variable (IV) when you added new variables to the regression equation?

b. Did the coefficient of that first, focal IV *decrease* in value? If so, this means the focal relationship is explained, in part, by some of these variables you added to the equation. In other words, the focal relationship is not the whole story; other factors affect, or influence, the association.

(continues)

TIP (*continued*)

TIP

c. Did that original variable (the focal IV) and the DV still maintain a *statistically significant* association? If so, the relationship remains valid, but may not be totally explained without the additional variables. If the focal relationship you tested in step 1, after adding new variables to the model, becomes nonsignificant (or "disappears,," statistically speaking), then you have a problem because the original focal relationship appears not to "hold" when you bring in other variables. This requires a "critical revisiting" of your theory, as Aneshensel would say, before you proceed with further analyses.

3. *Demonstrate that the focal relationship fits within an interlocking set of other relationships that are anticipated by the theory being tested, other relationships that are operationalized with antecedent, intervening, and consequent variable* (Aneshensel, 2002, p. 235). This step consists of elaborating, extending the focal relationship and "connecting the focal relationship to a network of other relationships" (p. 235). Your theory may have specified which factors are regarded as "antecedents to," which factors are "consequents to," and which factors might "intervene" in the focal relationship. In this step, you test what are the roles of all the variables your theory proposed:

   a. Do the variables show a relationship with the original IV (the one in the focal relationship)? If so, these are *antecedent* variables.

   b. Do the variables show a relationship with the original DV? If so, these might be *consequent* variables.

TIP

Antecedent and consequent-type variables do not affect the original focal relationship. They do affect the IV and the DV by themselves: The antecedent variables affect the focal IV, and the focal DV affects the consequent variables, like this:

$$\text{Antecedents} \rightarrow \text{IV}_{focal}$$
$$\text{DV}_{focal} \rightarrow \text{Consequents}$$

4. *Ascertain whether there are circumstances that modify the focal relationship and whether it applies uniformly to the entire population* (Aneshensel, 2002, p. 235). In this step, you are interested in learning whether the theoretical relationships you are testing through statistical analyses "hold" under various circumstances, groups, or situations. For instance, is the probability of the focal relationship happening still stronger than chance (statistically

significant) if you test it with your sample's girls then with the boys (for gender differences)? Or does the focal relationship change when you test the younger adolescents, then later test only the older adolescents? You need to test your data for these potential differences; hopefully your theory will offer suggestions of potential group differences that might be worth exploring.

QT5—Applying Theory to Secondary Data Analysis in Quantitative (Positivistic) Research

The term "secondary data" refers to information that you did not collect, data that you did not gather, yet is available for your use, courtesy of other researchers, or of tax-payers' dollars. Russell Schutt defines "secondary data analysis" as a "method of using preexisting data in a different way or to answer a different research question than intended by those who collected the data" (Schutt, 2006, p. 411). Surveys carried out with nationally representative samples (e.g., the General Social Survey, or GSS, the Adolescent Health survey, or ADDHEALTH survey) and funded by federal monies usually yield large datasets with numerous variables and, in some cases, data collected over many years (even decades). Russell Schutt's book titled *Investigating the Social World: The Process and Practice of Research* (2006) describes several sources of secondary data available to social scientists; many of these datasets contain variables of interest to public health scholars, too.

While the advantages of analyzing secondary data are numerous (including access to samples from which results can be inferred and generalized to the entire U.S. population), it is a form of research presenting important challenges. Some of these challenges relate to methodologic issues. For instance, as Schutt points out, with a secondary dataset, the analyst cannot test whether the data collection procedures were appropriate, and most certainly, he or she will not be able to engage in the iterative process of data-collection-and-refinement-of-research-questions. The potential mismatch between the research question the data analyst has in mind and the research question the original researchers proposed when the data were collected represents a thorny issue. More often than not, I hear from people conducting secondary data analysis the complaint that it's hard to "fit" their own questions onto answers designed to address *other, different* questions.

Especially "tricky" to handle—and I hesitate to say it this way, but it's true, it *is* "tricky"—is the issue of applying theory to this kind of data analysis. How should you proceed if this is the form of research you have chosen to conduct?

Guidelines and Tips: Applying Theory to Secondary Data Analysis

1. Learn as much as you can about the dataset's history.

> **TIP**
>
> Try to answer these questions specifically:
>
> a. What was the purpose in collecting the data?
> b. What did the measures (surveys, biological specimens, population records) intend to measure?
> c. When were the data collected (their historical context)?
> d. From whom were the data collected?
> e. By whom were they collected?
> f. How were they gathered?

2. Learn as much as you can about how the dataset has been used.

> **TIP**
>
> Search the published scientific literature—using the dataset's name as a search term—and identify all of the publications based on these data. Suggestions for which theories you might use might be in one of these publications.

3. Learn whether the survey was originally theory-based and upon which theory (or theories) the instrument was grounded. This information is crucial. If you learn that the survey was, in fact, associated with a given theory, you don't have to go any further, but learn about that theory and continue to use it as your roadmap for analysis.

4. If you learn the survey was not theory-based, you have two choices:

   a. To make *your* study a-theoretical and, therefore, suffer the consequences of what we discussed previously in the "a-theoretical research" section.

   b. To explore, within the data set, what might be some of the constructs being measured and which theory might aptly deal with these constructs and their relationships. For instance, let's imagine a given dataset contains seven questions that in your opinion appear to be measuring a person's self-efficacy. You might then test whether these seven items do, in fact, "hang together" and actually measure self-efficacy (statistical tests based on psychometrics theory will help you determine this). If the items do appear to measure self-efficacy and the dataset seems to contain more constructs related to self-efficacy (e.g., outcome expectations), you might think that perhaps invoking the help of Social Cognitive Theory may be helpful. After all, Social

Cognitive Theory presents a "road map" for how self-efficacy and outcome expectations might be related, and based on this road map, you can formulate hypotheses and test them statistically.

> **TIP**
>
> If you find the questions in the dataset don't seem to measure any "latent constructs" (constructs that have multiple dimensions and require more than one question to be measured adequately) and most questions are just prevalence-type questions (e.g., "Have you had the flu this year? How many people in your household had the flu?"), you may consider this a more epidemiological, descriptive study and not apply a theoretical framework.

QL—APPLYING THEORY TO QUALITATIVE (OR NATURALISTIC) RESEARCH

At a superficial level, we have come to think of qualitative research *negatively*. By the term "negative" I don't mean in a distorted, dismissive manner; I mean we normally define qualitative inquiry in terms of what it is *not*: Qualitative research is a type of inquiry that does *not* rely on numbers or statistics to tell the story of particular phenomena. It uses *words* or images to tell that story. I would argue, however, that such an understanding is not only simplistic, but reduces naturalistic inquiry so much that the image we create becomes an utter distortion. Qualitative research (also known as naturalistic inquiry) is quite a bit more than research that doesn't use numbers or the language of mathematics/statistics.

Norman Denzin and Yvonna Lincoln (2005) define qualitative research as

> . . . a situated activity that locates the observer in the world. It consists of a set of interpretive, material practices that make the world visible. These practices transform the world. They turn the world into a series of representations, including field notes, interviews, conversations, photographs, recordings, and memos to the self. At this level, qualitative research involves an interpretive, naturalistic approach to the world. This means that qualitative researchers study things in their *natural settings*, attempting to make sense of, or interpret, phenomena in terms of the meanings people bring to them. (p. 03)

Just as it was for quantitative inquiry, qualitative approaches to research are a way of seeing the world, of viewing science, and of approaching knowledge building. Qualitative researchers see the world in ways that oftentimes are quite opposite to the views of quantitative researchers. Primarily, qualitative research aims at understanding phenomena in its natural settings (hence, the label "naturalistic"), at telling in-depth stories of a phenomenon with "thick descriptions," vivid details, and enticing depictions. Quantitative research, on the other hand, seeks to generalize across settings, to uncover cause-and-effect relationships, and to predict (therefore, control) the phenomenon of interest. Think of the idea of "seeing the world differently" like this: Pretend two people, one from an Asian country and one from an African country, were asked to describe their experiences of spending one day at Disney World in the United States. How do you think each one would describe the same things: the rides, the parade on Main Street, the Disney characters, the music, and the food? If you were jotting down field notes, including what these two individuals said, you'd probably be surprised at the differences in their reports! Inevitably, each person would bring to his or her description a repertoire of words, expressions, names of colors, meanings of sounds, and appreciations of taste that would be quite unique and different from the other person's. Similarly, quantitative and qualitative researchers might focus on studying the same phenomenon; yet, after we read their studies, we sometimes think, "Which Disney World did *you* visit?"

Remember the five basic beliefs (or axioms) held by positivists? The five beliefs that shape positivists' view of science and knowledge building? Let's examine then the axioms of qualitative/naturalistic inquiry and think about how they compare to the positivistic ones. Such a comparison should help highlight how these two modes of research view things in completely different ways.

Here then are the basic beliefs/axioms of qualitative research (from pages 37 and 38 of Lincoln and Guba's, 1985, book *Naturalistic Inquiry*):

1. Beliefs regarding the nature of reality (ontology)—There are multiple constructed realities that can be studied only holistically; inquiry into these multiple realities will inevitably diverge (each inquiry raises more questions than it answers) so that prediction and control are unlikely outcomes although some level of understanding (*verstehen*) can be achieved.
2. Beliefs regarding the relationship of knower to known (epistemology)—The inquirer and the "object" or inquiry interact to influence one another; knower and known are inseparable.
3. Beliefs regarding the possibility of generalization—The aim of inquiry is to develop an idiographic [based on individual characteristics] body of knowledge in the form of "working hypotheses" that describe the individual case.
4. Beliefs regarding the possibility of causal linkages—All entities are in a state of mutual simultaneous shaping so that it is impossible to distinguish causes from effects.

5. Beliefs regarding the role of values in inquiry (axiology)—Inquiry is value-bound in at least five ways:
   a. Inquiries are influenced by *inquirer* values as expressed in the choice of a problem, evaluand, or policy option, and in the framing, bounding, and focusing of that problem, evaluand, or policy option.
   b. Inquiry is influenced by the choice of the *paradigm* that guides the investigation into the problem.
   c. Inquiry is influenced by the choice of the *substantive theory* utilized to guide the collection and analysis of data and in the interpretation of findings.
   d. Inquiry is influenced by the values that inhere in the *context*.
   e. With respect to . . . [points] a through d above, inquiry is either value-resonant (reinforcing or congruent) or value-dissonant (conflicting). (pp. 37–38).

QL1—The Role of Theory in Qualitative (Naturalistic) Research

Given these basic beliefs guiding qualitative research, what is the role theory might play in this paradigm? Well, first and foremost, notice what these axioms have to say about theory (in point 5.c, mentioned previously): that theory influences the inquiry. In other words, in contrast to the positivistic view that research is value neutral, qualitative researchers believe theories are not merely disinfected, sterile instruments one can "apply" to a research project, to generate hypotheses, determine the types of data to be collected, and help make sense of the statistical findings. Theories are living entities, rich with beliefs, values, and discourses, ready to influence the research process, but also to be influenced, altered, and reshaped by the research endeavor. In summary, theory plays a more dynamic role in qualitative research, moving beyond mere explanation (and prediction), to promoting critical social agendas, to *transforming* the world.

Naturalistic inquiry does not look to theory to provide a *foundation* for solving a problem or even for describing a particular problem. The naturalistic paradigm allows the researcher to use theory as a foundation, but only if he or she deems it is appropriate to do so or if grounding the study in a particular theoretical perspective is perceived as having an interpretive advantage. Most often, however, qualitative research will *not begin with theory*; it will allow theoretical propositions and explanations (the story) to emerge organically from the data, to surface from the individual stories told by many people who participate in a given study. In qualitative inquiry, researchers usually prefer to ground their *theory in the data*; in contrast, in quantitative inquiry, researchers prefer to ground their *data in the theory*.

Although qualitative research sees a role for theory that is more flexible than the one it enjoys in positivistic-type research, this does not mean that qualitative research is completely a-theoretical or that theory always emerges from the data. Because qualitative researchers do not approach a project as a completely "blank slate" and they do, in fact, bring a bundle of presuppositions, assumptions, and deeply held beliefs with them, we need to always remember that theoretical explanations are part of these presuppositions, assumptions, and beliefs. Because researchers have studied, before approaching a new research project, many different theories, have conducted related studies, and are knowledgeable of the different stories that can be told about a particular phenomenon, it is unrealistic to expect that they come to a research project, completely devoid of theory; therefore, at times, you will see qualitative researchers reporting their approach to the research project to include their theoretical perspectives. Here's an example of such reporting from a study conducted by Carolyn Clark (2001) entitled "Incarcerated Women and the Construction of the Self":

> [Clark begins by explaining to the readers the purpose of her study:]: I didn't set out to go to prison, at least not at first. My interest was in marginalized women and how they construct their sense of self. I was looking for women on the edges of society—not well educated, not well connected, not powerful in any of the ways we think about power, and certainly not visible. The prisons seemed an obvious place to begin. . . . Initially I framed my question in terms of women's identity development and its link to learning. . . . I found my theoretical ground in the literature on subjectivity, particularly approaches by feminists . . . working from postmodern and poststructural perspectives, who seek to understand how subjectivity is constructed within the complexities of social interaction and discourse. [After detailing the individual theories and theorists guiding her thinking, she concludes]: This is the theoretical framework that guides my thinking as I walk through the gates of the prison and come to know some of the women within. My goal is to gain an understanding of how these women construct their sense of self. As an adult educator, it is my hope that what I learn here will give me new insight into the process of personal or life-experience learning, and into the more complex process of transformational learning. (pp. 14–15)

QL2—Choosing a Theory (or Theories) for Your Qualitative Research Project

The guidelines and tips for *choosing* a theory for your qualitative study are, for the most part, the same ones I presented for quantitative research (so I won't bore you with useless repetitions, here); however, there are a few elements you must keep in mind.

Guidelines and Tips: Choosing a Theory for Your Qualitative Research Project

1. The *types* of theories you will employ in qualitative research might be of a very different kind than the ones you might apply in quantitative research. Because qualitative inquiry consists of multiple strategies and different approaches, the types of theories that will be invoked to frame the research will also vary. For example, while most theories used in quantitative-type research in health promotion will be those borrowed from the natural or the social sciences (e.g., biology or psychology), many of the theories used in qualitative research come from history, economics, political science, or even from studies of contemporary culture.

2. The *purpose of using* theory will also vary substantially according to the various qualitative strategies. For example, in the interepretivist or constructivist strategy, the purpose of theory is to facilitate description and understanding of the phenomenon from a particular perspective; in the critical theory strategy, theory is used to analyze the phenomenon from a historical, economical, or sociocultural "lens." In the deconstructivist strategy, theory is used for critique and for challenging the status quo. As you can see, none of these uses of theory center exclusively in identifying cause-and-effect relationships among factors in order to predict and control the phenomenon. These qualitative perspectives usually have an "agenda" to fulfill: critique of the social order, promotion of social justice, or challenges to the dominant discourses. Many of these agendas seek to understand and describe a phenomenon, yes (much like positivist-type research), but the use of theory in qualitative research goes *beyond* description, attempting to *transform* the world through the act of research, not merely to *observe* it. Theory in qualitative research, at times, does focus on cause-and-effect, but its spotlight usually moves *beyond* cause-and-effect to a more comprehensive understanding and to the promotion of social justice (Charmaz, 2005; Denzin & Lincoln, 2005).

QL3—Applying Theory to Qualitative Data Analysis and Interpretation

Applying theory to qualitative research in its many varieties is not as clear cut a process as the one for using theory in quantitative research. Why? Because qualitative researchers have the freedom to choose to begin their inquiry with theory to frame the study and its questions, or to bring theory into the study at the very end: when the researcher is ready to interpret the data. And to add to this potential complexity: Qualitative researchers may choose to *develop grounded theory*, i.e., let the theory emerge from the analysis of the data.

Guidelines and Tips: Applying Theory to Qualitative Data Analysis and Interpretation

1. First, understand the purpose of your qualitative project: Do you wish to develop theory or examine a given phenomenon?

2. If your purpose is to *develop theory* about a topic for which little-to-no-theory exists, then you should review the literature and document, as well as possible, the absence of a theory to explain the phenomenon in which you're interested.

3. If your purpose is to *develop theory*, when other theories already exist, you should invoke them—mainly for comparison purposes—at the latter stages of your work, during data interpretation. Present the currently available theories, explain how they have contributed to the scientific conversation about the topic, then compare your theory, the one you gleaned from analyzing your qualitative data to these other existing theories.

> **TIP**
> When comparing your theory to existing frameworks, stick to simple comparisons such as: which factors/constructs are similar between the theories? Which differ? What is the focal relationship in your theory as compared with other theories?

4. If the purpose of your study, however, is *not to develop theory*, you have to choose whether:

   a. You will bring an existing theoretical perspective to guide the development of your questions and the type of data you'll collect or

   b. You will "go directly" to your data collection, devoid of a theoretical frame (to avoid potentially biasing the data you'll be collecting) and later use theory to help analyze and interpret the data.

> **TIP**
> A very simple way (and simplistic, of course!) to think about these options is this: Where will theory show up in the write-up of your qualitative research? In (1) *the beginning* (like it does in most positivistic-type research), framing the questions and the type of data to be collected, or (2) in *the end* of the study (after data are presented) to help make sense of the findings?

5. If you choose to use theory to guide your study (option (1), above), the procedures will be similar to the ones employed in quantitative research: The theory will help you formulate the questions and determine the kind of data you must collect.

6. If you choose theory as a guiding framework, consider using it as a roadmap during data analysis also. For instance, theory can furnish the categories (based on the constructs and relationships it describes) for coding qualitative themes during a thematic analysis. Notice what Richard Boyatzis (1998) says about this in a book he wrote to teach qualitative researchers how to conduct thematic analysis of their data:

> A theme is a pattern found in the information [the data] that at the minimum describes and organizes possible observations or at the maximum interprets aspects of the phenomenon. . . . The themes may be initially generated inductively from the raw information or *generated deductively from theory* and prior research. (p. vii, emphasis mine)

7. If you choose not to use theory to guide the inquiry, then read Chapter 4 of Harry Wolcott's (2009) book *Writing Up Qualitative Research*. That chapter has the best treatment I've seen regarding how to link one's qualitative *findings* to theory. Because Wolcott distinguishes among three stages in qualitative data analysis—*description, analysis,* and *interpretation*—he argues, this way, about the use of theory:

> I urge you to hold off introducing theory until it is quite clear what you are interested in theorizing about and how that relates directly to what you have to report. . . . keep the *focus* on the descriptive task, until you have provided a solid basis for analysis and for determining where and how much to draw on the work of others. (p. 70)

Wolcott is clearly not a fan of using theory to guide the inquiry because whenever this is the purpose, what he has witnessed is far from theoretical guidance; in his words, "I have more often seen theory *imposed,* in a too-obvious effort to rationalize data already collected, than I have seen data collection guided by a theory already well in hand" (Wolcott, 2001, pp. 76–77); therefore, he prefers to see researchers bring theory to bear upon the *interpretation* phase of data analysis (if you want a better grasp of what Wolcott means by the differences among description, analysis, and interpretation, read his book *Transforming Qualitative Data: Description, Analysis, and Interpretation*). As Wolcott (2001) reminds us

> To whatever extent you intend to embrace theory, your interpretive passages [sometimes the discussion section in journal articles] are the place to draw in and draw upon it. This is far preferable to a premature and abstract discussion of theory offered by way of introduction. (p. 76)

8. When linking qualitative findings to theory, says Wolcott (2001), ". . . consider proposing multiple plausible interpretations rather than pressing single-mindedly for a particularly inviting one" (p. 76). In other words, consider interpreting your findings from different "places," from different theoretical perspectives: a feminist theory perspective versus an interpretivist perspective, for instance.

9. Be cautious. As Wolcott (2001) alerts

> Keep your theorizing modest and relevant. . . . Advancing theoretical knowledge is not a step that every researcher is prepared, or has been prepared, to make. Take your work as far as you are able. Point the way for others if you are not prepared to take the theoretical leap yourself, especially if and when it begins to *feel* like a leap, rather than making a pretense at doing the "theory thing." (p. 77)

QL4—Applying Theory to Secondary Data Analysis or Reanalysis of Qualitative Data

As it happens with quantitative data, oftentimes qualitative data sets become available for analyses. Many qualitative researchers, because their data are so rich (and there's usually so much of it!), quite often engage in reanalyses of their own data in order to answer new questions, different from the ones originally proposed.

The issues involved in applying theory to this kind of data analysis are similar to the ones we described for analyzing quantitative secondary data and the same ones that govern the use of theory in the analysis of primary data in qualitative research. There is really nothing to add here except a reminder that applying theory to secondary analysis of qualitative data might, in fact, be a bit less frustrating than attempting to "retro-fit" theory onto a quantitative data set. Because theory, in qualitative research, is viewed as a helpful tool, an added bonus for interpreting the data, qualitative researchers can tread lightly in their theory-linking efforts. Because in quantitative research theory is—more often than not—a *condition* for the study, it becomes tremendously frustrating to find a theory (and the question) that perfectly aligns itself with the answers provided in a secondary dataset.

QL5—Generating Theory in Qualitative Research

If the purpose of your qualitative research project centers on developing a theory about the phenomenon you're studying, then you would do best to familiarize yourself with grounded theory methods of data collection and analysis. According to Kathy Charmaz (2005),

> The term "grounded theory" refers both to a method of inquiry and to the product of inquiry. However, researchers commonly use the term to mean a specific mode of analysis. . . . Essentially, grounded theory methods are a set of flexible analytical guidelines that enable researchers to focus their data collection and to build inductive middle-range theories through successive levels of data analysis and conceptual development. . . . a grounded theory approach encourages researchers to remain close to their studied worlds and to develop an integrated set of theoretical concepts from their empirical materials that not only synthesize and interpret them but also show processual relationships. (pp. 507–508)

Many critics of grounded theory have had issues with the method's apparent "rigidity" and affinity for certain positivist assumptions and values (such as the importance of logic, analytical procedures, and beliefs about unbiased observers, says Charmaz, 2005). Nevertheless, the method has enabled researchers to develop and propose quite interesting theories. If employing a grounded theory perspective to your study seems attractive, the only guideline I offer here is a listing of some of the "classic" texts, as well as a few of the more contemporary treatments of the topic:

- Strauss, A., & Corbin, J. (1998). *Basics of Qualitative Research: Techniques and Procedures for Developing Grounded Theory.* Thousand Oaks, CA: Sage Publications.
- Charmaz, K. (2005). Grounded theory in the 21st century: applications for advancing social justice studies. In: N. K. Denzin, & Y. S. Lincoln (Eds.), *The SAGE Handbook of Qualitative Research* (3rd ed.). Thousand Oaks, CA: Sage Publications.
- Glaser, B. G. (1992). *Basics of Grounded Theory Analysis.* Mill Valley, CA: Sociology Press.
- To compare grounded theory to other qualitative traditions and to learn how to design qualitative studies using a grounded theory perspective, I recommend consulting: Creswell, J. W. (1998). *Qualitative Inquiry and Research Design: Choosing among Five Traditions.* Thousand Oaks, CA: Sage Publications.

MM—APPLYING THEORY TO MIXED METHODS (OR PRAGMATIST) RESEARCH

Mixed methods research (also referred to as mixed, multimethod, or pragmatist research) (Johnson, Onwuegbuzie, & Turner, 2007) has gained prominence in several fields of study in recent years. For many scholars, mixed methods research has achieved the status of "the third major research approach or research paradigm, along with qualitative research and quantitative research" (Johnson et al., 2007, p. 112).

Despite its newly found status, how to best define mixed methods research has been the focus of much debate. Burke Johnson, Anthony Onwuegbuzie, and Lisa Turner analyzed 19 different definitions of mixed methods research and, after consulting with several leaders in the field, provided a summary definition, or a "working definition," if you will (Johnson et al., 2007):

> Mixed methods research is the type of research in which a researcher or team of researchers combines elements of qualitative and quantitative research approaches (e.g., use of qualitative and quantitative viewpoints, data collection, analysis, inference techniques) for the broad purposes of breadth and depth of understanding and corroboration. (p. 123)

Mixed methods research carries the label "pragmatist" because its philosophical foundations can be found in the classic school of thought known as "pragmatism" (Johnson & Onwuegbuzie, 2004). Pragmatism, an eminently American philosophical movement, proposes that something is *true* only if it *works*. The movement, in its beginnings, attempted to offer very "down-to-earth" solutions to abstract, metaphysical debates. One of its main recommendations was for philosophers and theorists to examine the value of a theory in terms of its practical consequences or to "get in the habit of posing the following question: "*What concrete practical difference would it make if my theory were true and its rival(s) false?*" (McDermid, 2006).

Pragmatism, as it applies to social science research, tries to avoid fruitless debates over which of the previous paradigms (quantitative or qualitative) is superior for the purposes of social sciences research. The pragmatists' solution to the dilemma of which method is best, consists in reframing the issue: What matters is not which method is superior in and of itself, but which one is the most appropriate to answer specific questions to achieve a given study's objectives. Depending on the research question, a qualitative approach might work well, or yet, quantitative methods might represent a better fit. Whatever "works" to answer the research question: that's what is best or more valid—a very practical approach (for a helpful summary of the characteristics, strengths and weaknesses of Pragmatism, see Johnson & Ouwengbuzie, 2004, pp. 18 and 19).

The pragmatist research paradigm, according to Anthony Onwuegbuzie and Nancy Leech (2005), represents a fourth phase in the development of the social sciences. During the first phase, quantitative research—influenced by the tenets of positivism and the tools of mathematics and statistics—reigned supreme. The second phase brought forth qualitative research and the naturalistic paradigm, along with a sharp "polarization" between quantitative and qualitative approaches. The third phase emerged as a reaction to the negative criticisms being raised about social science research (in general); this phase saw the emergence of post-positivist research.

According to Onwuegbuzie and Leech (2005a), "post-positivism represented a compromise between the quantitative and qualitative research paradigms" (p. 269). Yet such compromise did not do much for *blending* the two paradigms. During the postpositivistic phase, while quantitative researchers began to concede there is no such thing as value-neutral/value-free research nor truly objective inquiry, many qualitative researchers still held on to the belief that qualitative methods are essentially incompatible with the quantitative worldview: "Arguing for the exclusive superiority of their qualitative orientation, they contended that these two paradigms could not and should not be mixed in any way" (Onwueg-buzie & Leech, 2005b, p. 270).

In the 1980s, the fourth phase in social science research emerged promoted by the pragmatists who believed that the two approaches could, in fact, coexist peacefully. Pragmatist researchers proposed that quantitative and qualitative methods are neither "mutually exclusive nor interchangeable" (p. 270) and that the "relationship between the quantitative and qualitative paradigms [consists] of isolated events lying on a *continuum* of scientific research" (Onwuegbuzie & Leech, 2005b, p. 270).

MM1—The Role of Theory in Mixed Methods Research

As we have seen in the previous sections, the application of theory to quantitative and qualitative research differs substantially: Quantitative research usually applies a deductive logic and tests theoretical propositions or hypotheses derived from a theory; in other words, it begins with theory, and the data collected either confirm or falsify that theory. Qualitative research applies an inductive logic and develops theoretical propositions from the data collected; in other words, developing theory is oftentimes the outcome of qualitative research, with the data collected furnishing the beginnings of that theory. Moreover, sometimes existing scientific theories are invoked by qualitative researchers to help interpret and understand the data.

So, with such disparate ways of using theory, you may be asking yourself: How can theory be used consistently throughout a mixed methods study? According to Carolyn Ridenour and Isadore Newman (2008), the "place of theory" in quantitative and qualitative research overlaps when one conducts a mixed method study (p. 29). To understand this overlap, it helps to see mixed methods as a *continuum* (Johnson & Onwuegbuzie, 2004):

> If you visualize a continuum with qualitative research anchored at one pole and quantitative research anchored at the other, mixed methods research covers the large set of points in the middle area. If one prefers to think categorically, mixed methods research sits in a new third chair, with qualitative research sitting on the left side and quantitative research sitting on the right side. (p. 15)

Within this continuum, mixed methods studies can be designed in at least nine different ways, according to Johnson and Owuengbuzie (2004), depending on the extent of blending and the sequence in which the different methods are employed. To be faithful to these designs, we would have to provide guidelines for applying theory to each one. Yet, in all honestly, we would gain little in doing so because the use of theory in each of the designs doesn't vary too much. It proves more useful and parsimonious, instead, to collapse these nine designs into broader, more encompassing categories and deal with these. For our purposes, then, I will provide guidelines for applying theory to mixed methods research of three kinds (three broader categories): Quantitative Dominant, Equal Status, and Qualitative Dominant (Johnson & Onwuegbuzie, 2004, p. 124).

Johnson et al. (2007) define these categories for us:

> Quantitative Dominant Mixed Methods Research . . . is the type of mixed research in which one *relies on a quantitative,* postpositivist view of the research process, while concurrently recognizing that the *addition of qualitative* data and approaches are likely to benefit most research projects.

> Qualitative Dominant Mixed Methods Research . . . *relies on a qualitative,* constructivist-postructuralist-crical view of the research process, while concurrently recognizing that the *addition of quantitative* data and approaches are likely to benefit most research projects.

> Equal Status Mixed Methods Research represents . . . *equal use of quantitative and qualitative approaches,* in a single research project. Both approaches are seen as making equally valid contributions to the insights to be gained from the research enterprise. (pp. 123–124, emphasis mine)

MM2—Choosing a Theory for Your Mixed Methods Research Project

Because mixed methods research combines quantitative and qualitative approaches and methods, choosing a theory for a mixed methods project will depend largely on the type of mixed methods study being conducted.

Guidelines and Tips: Choosing a Theory for Your Mixed Methods Research Project

1. Make sure you know which *type* of mixed methods research you will be using: equal status, qualitative dominant, or quantitative dominant.

TIP

To learn more about the types of mixed methods research, search for articles and books by these authors: Anthony Onwuegbuzie, Charles Teddlie, Abbas Tashakkori, R. Burke Johnson, and Nancy Leech.

2. If your study is quantitative dominant, follow the guidelines I proposed for choosing a theory for your quantitative research project.
3. If your study is qualitative dominant, follow the guidelines for choosing a theory for qualitative projects.
4. If your study is an equal status model, you will benefit from examining the guidelines for both the quantitative and qualitative projects.

MM3—Applying Theory to Mixed Methods Research

We would do well to keep in mind what Johnson and Ouwengbuzie say in their 2004 article as we handle the theories in mixed methods projects:

> . . . mixed-method designs are similar to conducting a quantitative mini-study and a qualitative mini-study in one overall research study. Nonetheless, to be considered a mixed-method design, the findings must be mixed or integrated at some point. (p. 20)

Guidelines and Tips: Applying Theory to Mixed Methods Research

1. Identify what type of mixed methods research your project will employ: equal status, quantitative dominant, or qualitative dominant.
2. Decide whether to have (1) a single theory or a set of theories that will apply to *both* the quantitative and the qualitative portions of the study or

(2) different—related and complementary—theories for the quantitative and qualitative portions.

3. Decide the sequence in which you will conduct the different portions of your study.

4. If you decide to *begin with the qualitative portion* (for exploratory purposes), you may apply the theory you develop, grounded in your data, to the quantitative (subsequent) portion of the study. For instance, you may decide to conduct several focus groups with adolescents to learn how they understand the concept of "healthy living." Based on the focus group qualitative data and the theoretical explanations that emerge from the data, you may then develop a survey instrument to assess how widespread those themes you encountered in the focus groups really are (by administering the survey to adolescents in various schools in your home state).

5. If you decide to *begin with the quantitative portion* (for hypotheses testing purposes), you may start with a strong, already-developed scientific theory, test your hypotheses, and then later use that same theory to help you analyze and interpret data from the qualitative (subsequent) portion of the study. For instance, you may wish to test whether young males' self-efficacy for using condoms during sexual intercourse predicts whether they will, in fact, use a condom in their next sexual encounter. You test this hypothesis with a large sample of college students by developing a theory-based survey instrument. Later, you invite students who completed your survey for an in-depth interview. Self-Efficacy Theory (Bandura, 1977), then, as it explains the dimensions, the constraints, and the factors affecting young adults' self-efficacy, may help you understand (and interpret) participants' perceptions of what might affect their confidence to use condoms.

6. In summary, when conducting mixed methods research, you may have the following scenarios take place (all of them, equally valid, don't forget!):

   a. The same theory for both the quantitative and the qualitative portions of the study

   b. Different theories for the quantitative and the qualitative portions of the study

   c. Theory "carryover" from the quantitative dominant portion into the qualitative portion

   d. Theory "carryover" from the qualitative dominant portion into the quantitative portion

SUGGESTIONS FOR PRACTICING THEORETICAL THINKING

1. Focus on a research project of your own, and test the guidelines provided in this chapter for choosing and applying theory to research.

2. Refine the guidelines by noting which ones work for you and which ones do not. Identify the procedures you implemented when the guidelines offered here did not work for you.

3. Besides yourself, have at least one of your colleagues attempt to use these guidelines. Discuss the strategies that were successful; develop new ones in place of the guidelines that didn't work for you. Share and compare experiences.

4. Mentor a junior colleague as he or she attempts to apply theory to a research project. As you teach these steps, they will be reinforced, and your comfort level with applying theory to research will increase.

Guidelines For Applying Theory—Checklists: Choosing a Theory

Choosing a Theory for a Quantitative or Qualitative Research Project

- ❑ 1. Name the problem/issue.
- ❑ 2. Conduct a brief search of the published literature related to the problem/issue/phenomenon.
- ❑ 3. Read articles identified during the search.
- ❑ 4. Note which theoretical framework each study employed (use a matrix).
- ❑ 5. Note the constructs and variables being examined in each study (use a matrix).
- ❑ 6. Examine matrix after having read 5 to 10 articles: Which theories are researchers currently using?
- ❑ 7. Identify potential "candidate theories."
- ❑ 8. Search reference sections of the articles read: Seek original citations for works describing candidate theories (books).
- ❑ 9. Read and learn about candidate theories.
- ❑ 10. Select the theory/theories to employ in the study.

Choosing a Theory for a Mixed Methods Research Project

- ❑ 1. Determine which type of mixed methods you will use: equal status, qualitative dominant, or quantitative dominant.
- ❑ 2. If study is quantitative dominant, follow guidelines for choosing a theory for a quantitative research project.

Choosing a Theory for a Mixed Methods Research Project

❏   3.   If study is qualitative dominant, follow guidelines for choosing a theory for a qualitative research project.

❏   4.   If study is equal status design, examine guidelines for both quantitative and qualitative research projects.

Guidelines for Applying Theory—Checklists: Grounding Research Questions and Hypotheses

Grounding Research Questions and Hypotheses in a Quantitative Research Project

❏   1.   Write a couple of paragraphs *naming* and *briefly describing* the theory you have chosen.

❏   2.   Write one paragraph identifying the theory's *main assumptions* and another paragraph presenting *your assumptions about the research topic.*

❏   3.   Identify, define, and explain (in writing) each of the factors you wish to examine in the study (provide conceptual and operational definitions).

❏   4.   Describe the relationships among the factors you chose to examine based on the theory's statements about these relationships.

❏   5.   Write your study's main research question and/or hypotheses.

❏   6.   Word each hypothesis as a relationship among the *numerical values* of your variables (expected differences, expected effects).

Guidelines for Applying Theory—Checklists: Applying Theory to Data Analysis

Applying Theory to Data Analysis in a Quantitative Research Project*

❏   1.   Assess whether the focal independent variable is associated with the dependent variable in the manner predicted by theory and at a level beyond chance.

❏   2.   Eliminate alternative explanations for the observed associations through the use of control and other independent variables.

❏   3.   Demonstrate that the focal relationship fits within an interlocking set of other relationships that are anticipated by the theory being tested and other relationships that are operationalized with antecedent, intervening, and consequent variables.

❏   4.   Ascertain whether there are circumstances that modify the focal relationship and whether it applies uniformly to the entire population.

   * Adapted from Aneshensel (2002, pp. 235)

Applying Theory to Secondary Data Analysis in a Quantitative Research Project

❏   1.   Learn about the dataset's history.

❏   2.   Learn how the dataset has been used.

❏   3.   Identify whether the data collection instrument was theory based (which theory?).

❏   4.   Choose whether to make your study a-theoretical, if the dataset was not theory based, or to explore the dataset for variables and constructs that might be explained by a given theory.

Guidelines for Applying Theory—Checklists: Applying Theory to Data Analysis

Applying Theory to Data Analysis and Interpretation in a Qualitative Research Project

☐   1. Determine the purpose of your qualitative project: theory development or other?

☐   2. Review the literature and document the absence of theory if purpose is to develop theory in the absence of theoretical frameworks.

☐   3. Invoke existing theory if purpose is to develop new theory. Compare and contrast your new theory to existing theories.

☐   4. Decide whether to use theory to guide the development of questions and methods or use theory to help analyze and interpret the data (will you use theory in the beginning or at the end of the study?).

☐   5. If choosing theory to guide study: see Guidelines for Grounding Research Questions and Hypotheses in a Quantitative Research Project.

☐   6. If choosing theory to analyze and interpret the data, consider using theoretical constructs for coding qualitative themes.

☐   7. If choosing theory to analyze and interpret data, read Chapter 4 of Harry Wolcott's book *Writing Up Qualitative Research* for detailed instructions on linking theory to interpretation of qualitative data.

☐   8. Consider interpret findings from more than one theoretical perspective.

☐   9. Be cautious: Keep theorizing modest and relevant.

Applying Theory to Secondary Data Analysis and Interpretation in a Qualitative Research Project

☐   Follow guidelines for applying theory to (primary) data analysis and interpretation in a qualitative research project (procedures are similar).

Guidelines for Applying Theory—Checklists: Applying Theory to Mixed Methods Research

Applying Theory to a Mixed Methods Research Project

☐   1. Identify the type of mixed methods research you will use: equal status, quantitative dominant, qualitative dominant.

☐   2. Decide between

      a. Having a single theory (or set of theories) for BOTH the quantitative and qualitative portions

      b. Having different (but related) theories for the quantitative and qualitative portions

☐   3. Decide the sequence to use in your study (quantitative or qualitative first?).

☐   4. Decide whether to "carry over" theory from the qualitative dominant portion into the quantitative portion of the study.

☐   5. Decide whether to "carry over" theory from the quantitative dominant portion into the qualitative portion of the study.

REFERENCES

Aneshensel, C. S. (2002). *Theory-Based Data Analysis for the Social Sciences*. Thousand Oaks, CA: Pine Forge Press.

Bandura, A. (1977). Self-efficacy: toward a unifying theory of behavioral change. *Psychological Review, 84*(2), 191–215.

Baron, R. M., & Kenny, D. A. (1986). The moderator–mediator variable distinction in social psychological research: conceptual, strategic, and statistical considerations. *Journal of Personality and Social Psychology, 51*(6), 1173–1182.

Boyatzis, R. E. (1998). *Transforming Qualitative Information: Thematic Analysis and Code Development*. Thousand Oaks, CA: Sage Publications.

Brewer, N. T., & Rimer, B. K. (2008). Perspectives on health behavior theories that focus on individuals. In K. Glanz, B. K. Rimer & K. Viswanath (Eds.), *Health Behavior and Health Education: Theory, Research, and Practice* (pp. 149–165). San Francisco: Jossey-Bass.

Charmaz, K. (2005). Grounded theory in the 21st century: applications for advancing social justice studies. In N. K. Denzin & Y. S. Lincoln (Eds.), *The SAGE Handbook of Qualitative Research* (3rd ed., pp. 507–535). Thousand Oaks: Sage Publications.

Clark, M. C. (2001). Incarcerated women and the construction of the self. In R. M. Cervero, B. C. Courtenay, & C. H. Monaghan (Eds.), *The Cyril O. Houle Scholars in Adult and Continuing Education Program Global Research Perspectives: Volume I* (pp. 14–27). Athens, GA: The University of Georgia.

Creswell, J. W. (1998). *Qualitative Inquiry and Research Design: Choosing Among Five Traditions*. Thousand Oaks: Sage Publications.

Denzin, N. K., & Lincoln, Y. S. (2005). Introduction: the discipline and practice of qualitative research. In N. K. Denzin & Y. S. Lincoln (Eds.), *The SAGE Handbook of Qualitative Research* (3rd ed., pp. 1–32). Thousand Oaks: Sage Publications.

Dressman, M. (2008). *Using Social Theory in Educational Research: A Practical Guide*. New York: Routledge.

Edberg, M. (2007). *Social and Behavioral Theory in Public Health*. Sudbury, MA: Jones and Bartlett Publishers.

Garrard, J. (2004). *Health Sciences Literature Review Made Easy: The Matrix Method* (2nd ed.). Sudbury, MA: Jones and Bartlett Publishers.

Glaser, B. G. (1992). *Basics of Grounded Theory Analysis*. Mill Valley, CA: Sociology Press.

Hayden, J. (2009). *Introduction to Health Behavior Theory*. Sudbury, MA: Jones and Bartlett Publishers.

Hochbaum, G. M., Sorenson, J. R., & Lorig, K. (1992). Theory in health education practice. *Health Education Quarterly, 19*(3), 295–313.

Johnson, R. B., & Onwuegbuzie, A. J. (2004). Mixed methods research: a research paradigm whose time has come. *Educational Researcher, 33*(7), 14–26.

Johnson, R. B., Onwuegbuzie, A. J., & Turner, L. A. (2007). Toward a definition of mixed methods research. *Journal of Mixed Methods Research, 1*(2), 112–133.

Lincoln, Y., & Guba, E. G. (1985). *Naturalistic Inquiry*. Newbury Park, CA: Sage Publications.

McDermid, D. (2006). *The Internet Encyclopedia of Philosophy: Pragmatism*. Available from www.iep.utm.edu/p/pragmati.htm#H2

MICRA Inc. (1991, April 2002). *Roget's Thesaurus of English Words and Phrases*. Available from http://poets.notredame.ac.jp/Roget/

Onwuegbuzie, A. J., & Leech, N. L. (2005a). On becoming a pragmatic researcher: the importance of combining quantitative and qualitative research methodologies. *International Journal of Social Research Methodology, 8*(5), 375–387.

Onwuegbuzie, A. J., & Leech, N. L. (2005b). Taking the "Q" out of research: teaching research methodology courses without the divide between quantitative and qualitative paradigms. *Quality & Quantity, 39*, 267–296.

Ridenour, C., & Newman, I. (2008). *Mixed Methods Research: Exploring the Interactive Continuum.* Carbondale, IL: Southern Illinois University Press.

Schutt, R. K. (2006). *Investigating the Social World: The Process and Practice of Research* (5th ed.). Thousand Oaks, CA: Sage Publications.

Shoemaker, P. J., Tankard Jr., J. W., & Lasorsa, D. L. (2004). *How to Build Social Science Theories.* Thousand Oaks, CA: Sage Publications.

Strauss, A., & Corbin, J. (1998). *Basics of Qualitative Research: Techniques and Procedures for Developing Grounded Theory* (2nd ed.). Thousand Oaks, CA: Sage Publications.

Wolcott, H. F. (1994). *Transforming Qualitative Data: Description, Analysis, and Interpretation.* Thousand Oaks: Sage Publications.

Wolcott, H. F. (2001). *Writing Up Qualitative Research* (2nd ed.). Thousand Oaks: Sage Publications.

Wolcott, H. F. (2009). *Writing Up Qualitative Research* (3rd ed.). Thousand Oaks: Sage Publications.

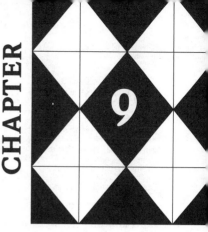

Applying Theory to Program Planning and Evaluation

Learning Objectives

When you finish reading this chapter, you will be able to:

1. List the advantages of using theory to develop health promotion programs.

2. Explain the concept of implicit theories, or theories of action (or why health promotion programs are never completely a-theoretical).

3. Name two prominent models that facilitate an "ideal" application of theory to program planning.

4. Identify "real-world" strategies for using theory in program planning.

5. Describe two ways in which theory can be relevant for program evaluators.

6. List the characteristics of evaluations aimed at theory testing and of those focused on assessing programs' effectiveness.

7. Explain why program evaluation can be viewed as a form of theoretical thinking.

THEORY AND PRACTICE

If you have been reading the book from the beginning, it may have already crossed your mind that the phrase "applying theory to practice" is redundant. As we saw in Chapter 1, theory *is* a form of practice. Because theorizing involves asking certain types of questions, questioning the status quo, seeking the most plausible and meaningful answers, and building a narrative or logical structure for the questions and their answers, theory is a form of "action." It *does* all of these things; therefore, to use the phrase "apply theory to practice" is akin to saying "apply theory to theory" or "apply practice to practice." It makes little sense if you think about it.

Yet there is a dimension of the public health profession that requires we develop, implement, and evaluate interventions, or programs. This is the "bread-and-butter" of health promotion, and when we talk about theory, we do refer to applying theory to health promotion programming and evaluation as "applying theory to practice." So, let's maintain the phraseology (even if redundant) and ask the very practical question, "*How does one go about 'applying theory' when planning or evaluating a health promotion program?*"

The answer is not simple, as you might expect. There is no quick-and-easy set of strategies one can apply to bring theory to a program or to its evaluation, and practitioners have little, if any, time to engage in one more intricate task; after all, they work in an applied field, and there are so many complicated issues to attend to already, so many fires to put out, so many health problems to solve. A very common complaint practitioners have is lack of time to accomplish everything on their "to-do" lists. Who has time to sit back and *theorize* about things, especially if theory always seems so complex, so abstract, so technical? The authors of the book *Health and Modernity: The Role of Theory in Health Promotion*, David McQueen and his colleagues (2007), acknowledge this reality of health promotion practice, based on their own experiences in the field:

> It has often been said that there is nothing as practical as a good theory, a phrase attributed to Kurt Lewin (1951) and as a statement it reflects our views. During our public health careers most of us have been involved in work that is applied and often carried out with a heavy emphasis on how we are going to carry out an intervention. In fact, considerable time is often devoted to the nuts and bolts of a project, for example, how to conduct a survey, how to interview, how to engage the community and so on. In the excitement of the day to day challenges one often has little time to examine the theoretical underpinnings of a project, let alone go into a deeper reflexive discourse on why one is doing it. (pp. 2–3)

THE ROLE OF THEORY IN PROGRAM PLANNING

Given the applied nature of health promotion, the complexity inherent in applying theory, and the daily realities faced by practitioners, the question then becomes: "Why should practitioners even *care* about theory?" In Chapter 2, we discussed some answers to this question; there, I proposed several reasons why theory has important contributions to make to health promotion practice. While I won't repeat those arguments here, I urge you to remember, however, what happens when we engage in a-theoretical research (see the previous chapter). With the reasons listed in Chapter 2 and the a-theoretical research scenario from Chapter 8 in mind, ask yourself: what might a-theoretical program planning and evaluation look like?

At the very minimum, it will lead to programs and interventions that are "unexamined and underevaluated," to a nonreflexive practice (McQueen et al., 2007, p. 3), and at worst, to constant "re-inventing of the wheel," as Hochbaum, Sprenson, and Lorig (1992) point out:

> Health education, as every profession, must deal with an infinite variety of problems, situations, challenges. . . . These challenges could become overwhelming if each problem and each problem situation were so unique that we would have to search for new solutions every time. Luckily, there are always some common elements, factors, or variables that arise and exert themselves in many apparently dissimilar problem situations. . . . Theories aim at identifying and helping us understand elements that affect seemingly diverse classes of behaviors and tell us how these elements function. They may also suggest or actually offer ideas of how we can influence such elements under a variety of circumstances and thereby furnish us with valuable tools for solving a wide variety of problems in our work. (pp. 295–296)

Therefore—much as in the case of research—theory has a very important *practical* role to play in planning health promotion interventions and their evaluations. Thus, choosing to ignore theory has a cost, as Hochbaum and his colleagues remind us: It "robs practitioners of potentially useful tools," and "it inhibits the emergence of novel approaches to problems. As Pasteur said, "Theory is the mother of practice. Without theory, *practice is just routine born of habit*" (Hochbaum et al., 1992, p. 296, emphasis mine).

Having admitted that theory plays an important and practical role in program planning and evaluation and that a-theoretical interventions suffer from tremendous limitations, I would be remiss if I didn't remind you of something else you may have learned by now: Such a perspective is limited to the notion of theory as *scientific* theory. All that was previously said about the important and practical role theory plays in health promotion programming and evaluation presupposes that by *theory* we mean social science or behavior change theories.

If, however, we assume a broader approach to theory (theory as sense-making, as story telling—the approaches we discussed in Chapter 1), we conclude there is no such thing as an a-theoretical program ever. All programs are based on an internal logic on a story that recounts past successes, recasts previous failures, and explains how to reach the finish line: the outcomes the program proposes to achieve. A common difficulty we sometimes have is not being able to "see" this internal logic, to identify the stories practitioners are telling about their programs. Both stories and logic are often not explicitly articulated by the program planners and staff. Here's how McQueen et al. (2007) pose the issue:

> We would argue that health promotion practice has always possessed theoretical underpinnings, just not explicit. That is, there is always an underlying episte-mology behind actions even when they are not explicitly stated, even when they are not fully understood by the practitioner, and even where the practitioners would state that they operate with no theoretical base. (2007, p. 3)

The reality that programs are never completely devoid of theory, even if their planners do not invoke any of the traditional health promotion theories came to life for me during the evaluation I conducted between 2000 and 2005—which I briefly mentioned in Chapter 3. The evaluation comprised the assessment of various programs (for children and adolescents) focused on promoting abstinence from sexual activity before marriage. The programs were funded by federal dollars channeled through the state of Texas. In order to obtain funding, the programs had to submit a grant proposal to the Texas Department of State Health Services. Part of the evaluation plan my research team and I developed involved carefully examining each of the programs' submitted proposal: We needed to learn which outcomes programs wished to achieve and which activities they had planned, among other factors. We also searched the proposals to determine which health promotion theories were being used. To our dismay, of the 32 grant proposals we examined, only two claimed to base their programs on behavior change theories. One program mentioned the Risk-Protective Factor Model and the other Social Cognitive Theory along with Diffusion of Innovations Theory (Goodson, Pruitt, Suther, Wilson, & Buhi, 2006).

Yet, despite such lack of scientific theoretical grounding, it became clear to our team, in the course of the evaluation, that each of these programs had a story to tell—a story that included notions of cause and effect that explained why program planners had chosen one activity over another. Later, we concluded, those stories resembled the ones told by the scientific theories and the research evidence. If you recall the example I gave in Chapter 3, one of the programs articulated an extremely coherent explanation of why a group dance activity for middle-school girls could lead to sexually abstinent behavior (because the dance group had the potential to influence girls' self-esteem; increased self-esteem was seen as a protective factor for sexual risk-taking). As we (Goodson et al., 2006) wrote in an article describing these programs' implicit theories,

> This [evaluation's] findings indicate that abstinence-only-until-marriage programs in this Texas sample employed a plethora of activities to deliver the abstinence message to youth. Although most of the programs (with only two exceptions) were not based on scientific theories of adolescent development or behavior change theories, our findings suggest that the staff members from these programs are able to articulate a cogent set of propositions to explain how their program's activities lead to abstinent behavior among program participants. Moreover, the articulations uncovered in our sample were—in large part—consistent with empirical and theoretical data on nonsexual antecedents of adolescent sexual behavior. (pp. 267–268)

The take-home point here is this: When we critique programs and interventions for not employing health promotion or behavior change theories, our critique presupposes a limited, restricted idea of theory: theories as scientific propositions. Yet we would do well to keep in mind that programs always do, in fact, employ theory: theories as sets of specific questions and answers that make sense out of the practical reality addressed by the programs. All programs come wrapped up in these sets of questions; therefore, all programs are theory based.

APPLYING THEORY TO PROGRAM PLANNING

Because there is plenty of evidence supporting the notion that programs that are, in fact, based on scientific theories perform better than those that aren't (see Chapter 3), it remains a professional and practical duty to address the question: "*How does one apply scientific theories to program planning and evaluation?*" While detailed descriptions of the processes involved in tying theory to *research* appear sparsely in the health promotion literature, fortunately, procedures for applying theory to program planning and evaluation abound. For this reason, I keep my writing about this topic brief (now, aren't you *thankful!*).

Another reason I wish to write less in this chapter has to do with my own experience: I have extensive experience in thinking theoretically within my research projects and program evaluations; I have much less experience developing health promotion programs. Thank my inexperience then for having a shorter chapter to read here; however, I do want to provide you with some "pointers," places to go where you will find step-by-step procedures both for program planning and evaluation. I will not, however, present these "pointers" as sets of guidelines as I did in the previous chapter; you will find such guidelines in the materials I recommend to you here.

To begin our discussion about using theory to plan a program, it's important to keep this simple notion in mind: When it comes to strategies for grounding a health promotion intervention in behavior change (or other types of) theories, practitioners oftentimes describe the process as consisting primarily of two mutually exclusive options: (1) the "ideal" strategy and (2) the "real-world" strategy. Let's consider each of these two strategies, carefully.

Applying Theory to Program Planning: The "Ideal" Strategy

Ideally, looking to theory for help in developing a sound intervention begins very early in the planning process: Planners identify the outcomes they wish the program to achieve and work "backward." This backtracking procedure involves determining which factors contribute to that outcome. For example, let's imagine a state health department wishes to improve the levels of flu vaccinations among older low-income adults. Program planners, therefore, begin by identifying the desired outcome, or the goal of the intervention: increase the number of flu vaccinations among older, low income adults by 30% this year.

After the outcome is identified, the next step usually consists of determining which factors influence whether low income adults get or don't get immunized. Program planners, at this stage, have a couple of options. One of them is to examine previously collected data the health department may have and see whether those data provide any "clues" as to what might be keeping this population group from obtaining a flu shot each year.

The "ideal" option, however, is to allow theory to provide these explanations of which factors might explain immunization behavior and to determine which ones the current program can reasonably address. If program planners are familiar with some of the health promotion theories, they might think of the Health Belief Model as a good candidate. The Health Belief Model was developed to help professionals in the U.S. Public Health Service identify reasons why people were not obtaining free tuberculosis screening in the mid 1950s (Champion & Skinner, 2008). The model proposes that people only become motivated to submit to testing if they perceive the disease to be serious, if they see themselves as being at risk for this serious disease, and if there are no deterrents, or barriers, to getting the test (in other words, if it's convenient and few obstacles are present). The model also proposes that all these factors come into play *synergistically*; in other words, focusing on only one factor (e.g., perceived severity) may not lead to the desired outcome.

If program planners decide the Health Belief Model tells a story adequate enough to explain the issue of flu vaccination, they may choose to ground their program in this model. If they pick the model, then they must decide which factors might be the ones most likely to explain what's going on with flu shots among *their* target population. Let's say they identify that for this group of people the main issue is access to free vaccines. Therefore, making free vaccines available could be an outcome of the program. Yet, because having free vaccines won't guarantee people will get them, an educational campaign, designed specifically for that group, will be needed. And the campaign should tailor its message to address people's perception of how serious it can be to get the flu at advanced ages (perceived severity), as well as how susceptible to contracting the flu, older people can become (perceived susceptibility).

So, how does this "ideal" approach differ from an a-theoretical approach? Without the assistance of a model or theory (in our example, the Health Belief Model), program planners would be at a loss regarding which factors to address, which elements to "correct" in the system, which messages to provide to people. Planning would rely on professionals' past experiences with similar programs (what worked in the past is bound to work again!) or on these professionals' preferences for how things should be done. It should be apparent to you that this alternative is very likely to fail, precisely because it's relying mostly on chance. It *may work* (by chance), but it certainly will not work as *efficiently* as it could.

Fortunately, the "ideal" strategy—although the term sounds incredibly "lofty" and out of reach, it really isn't—has been carefully described by prominent scholars in the field, and their step-by-step processes are readily available. I'm referring specifically to two planning models that provide detailed specifications of how to apply behavior (and other types of) theories to planning health promotion interventions: the PRECEDE–PROCEED model and Intervention Mapping (Bartholomew, Parcel, Kok, & Gottlieb, 2006; Green & Kreuter, 2005).

One "Ideal" Strategy: The PRECEDE–PROCEED Model

In the current edition of the Glanz book, Chapter 18 addresses precisely this issue: Using the PRECEDE–PROCEED Model to Apply Health Behavior Theories (Gielen, McDonald, Gary, & Bone, 2008). The authors acknowledge the model has "been a cornerstone of health promotion practice for more than three decades" (p. 408) and describe it as a *road map* guiding intervention development: "[The PRECEDE] acronym stands for Predisposing, Reinforcing, and Enabling Constructs in Educational/Environmental Diagnosis and Evaluation. PRECEDE is based on the premise that, just as medical diagnosis precedes a treatment plan, so should educational diagnosis precede an intervention plan" (Gielen et al., 2008, p. 409).

Developed in the 1970s, the model has undergone two major revisions: one in 1991 and one in 2005. The 1991 revision added the PROCEED portion of the model as we now know it: Policy, Regulatory, and Organizational Constructs in Educational and Environmental Development. For Andrea C. Gielen and her co-authors, this addition tried to meet the growing "importance of environmental factors as determinants of health and health behaviors" (p. 409). The 2005 revision recognizes—more strongly than the previous versions—the "growing interest in ecological and participatory approaches" (p. 409) to health promotion and adds genetic factors to the behavioral and environmental determinants previously in place (Green & Kreuter, 2005).

The PRECEDE–PROCEED Model takes us through the entire process of developing, implementing, and evaluating health promotion interventions, navigating across eight distinct phases: (1) social assessment, (2) epidemiological assessment, (3) educational and ecological assessment, (4) administrative and policy assessment and intervention alignment, (5) implementation, (6) process evaluation, (7) impact evaluation, and (8) outcome evaluation (Green & Kreuter, 2005). Health promotion (and other social, economic, and biological) theories can play a guiding role in each of these phases: If the PRECEDE–PROCEED model functions as a road map, the theories offer specific *directions* to a destination, say Gielen et al. (p. 408).

Although neither the authors of the model nor Gielen and her chapter co-authors attempt to specify which theories are applicable in which phase, they offer important suggestions for which *types* of theories might be applicable at each point. For instance, when discussing application of theory to Phase 1 (Social assessment), Gielen and colleagues remind us that "at this phase in the program planning process, community organizing theories and principles are relevant" (p. 411); when discussing theory in Phase 2 (epidemiological assessment), they write, "Interpersonal theories of behavior change can be useful at this stage of the PRECEDE–PROCEED framework because of the emphasis on the interaction between individuals and their environment" (p. 414); when writing about Phase 3 (Educational and ecological assessment), the authors state, "All three levels of change theories—individual, interpersonal, and community—can be useful at this stage of the planning process" (p. 415). So, although the PRECEDE–PROCEED model does not offer practitioners specific suggestions of which theories to choose in each phase, it contains recommendations for which *levels* of theories should be considered at each step.

Another "Ideal" Strategy: Intervention Mapping

Another important tool to assist program planners in developing a theory-based program, step-by-step, is Intervention Mapping. Developed more recently than the PRECEDE–PROCEED model (in the 1980s), the purpose of Intervention Mapping is "to provide health education program planners with a framework for effective decision making at each step in intervention, planning, implementation, and evaluation" (Bartholomew et al., 2006, p. 3). The model consists of six steps. Each step outlines a complete set of tasks. In summarized form, these are the six steps and related tasks (pp. 15–22):

Step 1: Conduct a needs assessment or problem analysis
Tasks:
- Plan needs assessment with PRECEDE model
- Assess health, quality of life, behavior, and environment
- Asses capacity
- Establish program outcomes

Step 2: Create matrices of change objectives based on the determinants of behavior and environmental conditions.
Tasks:
- State expected changes in behavior and environment
- Specify performance objectives
- Specify determinants
- Create matrices of change objectives

Step 3: Select theory-based intervention methods and practical strategies.
Tasks:
- Review program ideas with interested participants
- Identify theoretical methods
- Choose program methods
- Select or design strategies
- Ensure that strategies match change objectives

Step 4: Translate methods and strategies into an organized program.
Tasks:

- Consult with intended participants and implementers
- Create program scope, sequence, theme, and materials list
- Develop design documents and protocols
- Review available materials
- Develop program materials
- Pretest program materials with target groups and implementers and oversee materials production

Step 5: Plan for adoption, implementation, and sustainability of the program.
Tasks:

- Identify adopters and users
- Specify adoption, implementation, and sustainability performance objectives
- Specify determinants and create matrix
- Select methods and strategies
- Design interventions to affect program use

Step 6: Generate an evaluation plan
Tasks:

- Describe the program
- Describe program outcomes and effect questions
- Write questions based on matrix
- Write process questions
- Develop indicators and measures
- Specify evaluation designs

As you can read in the outline above, Intervention Mapping consists of well-defined tasks and action steps program planners can carry out when planning a program. Additionally, Intervention Mapping authors make it a point to discuss the use of behavioral, environmental, and other types of theory as conceptual guides at each of these steps.

When addressing the use of behavioral or environmental theories, the guidelines offered in Intervention Mapping for choosing theoretical frameworks are very similar to those I proposed for selecting a theory for a quantitative research project (in Chapter 8). A major difference between my guidelines for research and the Intervention Mapping process lies in the emphasis Intervention Mapping places on selecting intervention *methods* from the theories, too. In other words, the model emphasizes learning from theory not only which factors influence or alter health behaviors but also *how to* affect or influence these factors.

I won't present here the details of the procedures proposed by Intervention Mapping—for that, the authors of the model have written a book, which I highly recommend, if you're interested in having a useful and practical tool at hand. The book is called *Planning Health Promotion Programs: an Intervention Mapping Approach* and was written by L. Kay Bartholomew, Guy S. Parcel, Gerjo Kok, and Nell H. Gottlieb (Dr. Gottlieb was my faculty mentor during my PhD training at The University of Texas at Austin). The process, the steps, and the tasks offered by Intervention Mapping are invaluable, yet complex. The authors themselves acknowledge that grounding a program on available theory and evidence is quite technical, and therefore, their text attempts to describe each step in as much practical detail as possible (Bartholomew et al., 2006):

> Sometimes the processes involved in understanding a problem or answering a question with empirical data and theory are complex and time consuming. Many health educators do not persevere through the difficulties. Consequently understanding often is incomplete or inadequate, and intervention is faulty. Therefore, we provide considerable detail about how to undertake these core processes. (p. 36)

Applying Theory to Program Planning: The "Real World" Strategy

Structures and strategies to facilitate the "ideal" incorporation of theory into the planning of health promotion programs—such as PRECEDE–PROCEED and Intervention Mapping—have been well defined, are readily available, and have stood the test of time: They *work*. Nevertheless, my own conversations with practitioners reveal few of them have the time, the interest, or perhaps the training to even remember to "go back to basics" when their bosses charge them with developing a campaign to improve flu vaccinations; a campaign that, by the way, needs to begin in two weeks, requires evaluation findings be ready three months from now, and the budget rules only allow spending money to develop a media campaign. . . . You get the picture: While the "boss" also operates under significant constraints, she seems to ignore the fact the practitioner she charged with developing the program has no staff available to help with planning and only one part-time assistant to help with clerical tasks. That's reality for many health departments and services, nationwide (and internationally, too).

Another "reality" I've heard practitioners talk about is the one I mentioned in Chapter 3: Personnel who write grants to obtain funding for a program will quite often write a proposal outlining a theory-based program. In the proposal, they will explain the theories grounding the program and how these theories inform the choice of methods and strategies the program will implement. After the grant is awarded, however, program staff ignore the grant and its proposed plan and revert to "business as usual," choosing program activities based on personal preferences, past experiences, and expertise. (Remember my conversation with the grant author who admitted he wrote theory into a proposal just to "push the buttons" of the funding agency? See Chapter 3). It isn't difficult to understand this practice: Public health personnel have little time to think, much less think *theoretically* about, or reflect on, their daily practice. So, how can theory be brought into play, within these contextual, but very real, limitations?

If the "ideal" program development strategies begin by searching for theoretical determinants or factors that influence the outcome the program wishes to achieve, the "real" strategies, more often than not, begin with the constraints placed upon program planners: the amount of money allocated to their program, the need to choose among priorities (given the money will not allow to address *everything* the "boss" wants addressed), and the need to choose strategies that have proven effective in similar programs. What can practitioners do then to bring any kind of theoretical reflection to the process? How can their programs be theory based or, more realistically, loosely coupled with theory to improve their chances of effectiveness?

Developing a Program's Implicit Theory

On a small whiteboard that hangs in the hallway leading to my office at Texas A&M University, someone recently wrote: "Acknowledge. Move on." I confess I have mixed feelings when I walk past that board: At times, I think, "How rude! Telling people to just move on. . . . One has no idea what serious problems people might be dealing with, what deep-seated pain they may have building in their hearts, what need for comforting words and gestures . . . and the only motivation this saying can offer is to move on?!" At other times, my mind tells me: "Yes, undoubtedly, the best strategy in all of life is to acknowledge and move on. Nothing healthier."

Despite the feelings you might experience if you, too, saw this statement each time you walked to your office, definitely, the first "moment" in planning a program in the "real" world is the one in which the program team acknowledges the constraints imposed on them and moves on(ward). If lobbying for changes, negotiating more funding, requesting added flexibility for using the funds, and asking for more time to prepare a better quality evaluation—if all these are reasonable to do—then they should be attempted before acknowledging and moving on. Program planners in the "real" world, however, often have little recourse and must attend to their tasks as they have been defined for them.

Whatever the constraints placed on program planners might be preventing them from developing a theory-based plan, there is still one thing they *can* do. They can reserve a couple of hours of planning to spell out, write down, or even graph the logic underlying their proposed plan (Donaldson, 2007). Even a bulleted list of items, which could be identified after a brainstorming session with the program's planning team, could help to identify the logic (and, if there's time and motivation, the *assumptions*) guiding the program. Let's return to our flu vaccination program. The goal is to increase the rates of flu vaccinations among older low-income adults in Silver City. The budget is limited and can only be spent on a media campaign. Free vaccinations are available but can only be provided at the main headquarters of Silver City's health department (which happens to be located downtown).

Based on this scenario, program planners might develop a rudimentary graph of the theory of action underlying their program, thus far. What the graph in Figure 9–1 shows is this: program staff will develop a media campaign they hope will increase the rates of flu vaccination among older low-income adults in Silver City.

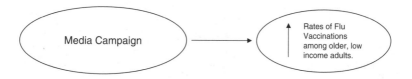

FIGURE 9–1 Graphic Representation of Flu Vaccine Campaign

As discussions about which messages to communicate in the media campaign evolve, however, some planners may have their own notions of which messages might be more effective. "We could send the message that older adults are more susceptible to contracting the flu, during the winter season, and the flu shot can protect both them and other susceptible populations," says one member of the planning team.

Now, program planners can graph the logic that's taking shape in their program, this way (Figure 9–2):

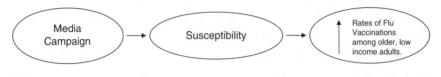

FIGURE 9–2 Graphic Representation of Underlying Logic for Flu Campaign

Let's imagine some planners become concerned, however, with focusing on the message of susceptibility to the flu. They wonder if this notion might scare the older adult population and instead of stirring them to action might immobilize them through fear. Another planner suggests then that the message of susceptibility could remain central to the campaign, but should be counterbalanced by another equally forceful message: that older adults can, in fact, do something about this increased risk. They are capable of taking charge of their own health; they can get vaccinations this season. And if they can come to the health department, those vaccinations will cost them nothing. The entire planning team agrees with the idea, and now the graph of the program's logic should look something like what is shown in Figure 9–3.

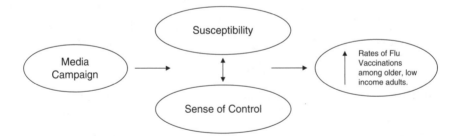

FIGURE 9–3 Graphic Representation of Program Logic (implicit theory) for Flu Campaign

After a rudimentary logic structure is outlined or graphed (no need for extensive planning documents; a graph similar to the ones you just saw, drafted during brainstorming sessions, might suffice), planners are able to use this "picture" as a roadmap for their program. What's even more interesting: After the underlying logic of the program is documented, it can easily be checked against the available literature for validation. A health department intern, or someone with fewer responsibilities in the team, can be asked to search the literature for documentation of programs similar to the one being developed. The person doing the search can easily use the key words appearing in the graph as search terms. Another person could be responsible then for scanning the identified literature and checking whether the program planning team is on the right track with their ideas: whether other studies have found evidence that focusing media campaigns on susceptibility and sense of control (or self-efficacy) can, in fact, influence (in this case, increase) vaccination uptake behaviors. During these literature searches and checks, one may find that adding other related messages might increase the effectiveness of the campaign. For instance, addressing people's perceptions of the barriers they have to overcome to obtain the free vaccine might be a useful theme to consider. Examples of these barriers might be obtaining transportation to go downtown, having to go to the health department or to a pharmacy alone, and not knowing who to ask whether the vaccine might interfere with current medications.

Having a roadmap of the program's implicit theory (theory of action or "espoused theory") will facilitate the implementation process because, as logical connections are made clear, most of the "guess work" related to where the program should focus its efforts will be gone. The roadmap allows efforts to be more focused, less scattered, and less reliant on chance. The roadmap also will be of tremendous help to program evaluators later in the evaluation process (as we discuss later in this chapter). As Patton (1997) appropriately stated, "The purpose of thoroughly delineating a program's theory of action is to assist practitioners in making explicit their assumptions about the linkages between inputs, activities, immediate outputs, intermediate outcomes, and ultimate goals" (p. 225).

Notice that, in uncovering the implicit theory in our sample program, none of the common behavior change or health promotion theories were invoked or discussed. For those of you familiar with these theories, however, you might easily have recognized the implicit logic in our example deals with constructs from Social Cognitive Theory (sense of control or self-efficacy) and from the Health Belief Model (perceived susceptibility). If the more curious among the program's team members then wish to ask the theoretical question—"*Under which circumstances does perceived susceptibility lead people to take preventive action?*"—then a foray into the theories themselves, to better understand the mechanisms underlying the logical relationships, can be undertaken. Yet, for developing a program's theory of action, espoused or implicit theory, one need not *begin* with scientific theories; one can start with telling the program's *story*.

THE ROLE OF THEORY IN PROGRAM EVALUATION

Although the notion of evaluation is intuitive and self-explanatory, it may be helpful to revisit a definition of *program evaluation* to make sure we have the same concepts in mind when using the phrase. Emil Posavac and Raymond Carey (2007) (authors of a textbook I often use when teaching Health Program Evaluation courses) define the terms this way:

> Program evaluation is a collection of methods, skills, and sensitivities necessary to determine whether a human service is needed and likely to be used, whether the service is sufficiently intensive to meet the unmet needs identified, whether the service is offered as planned, and whether the service actually does help people in need at a reasonable cost without unacceptable side effects. Utilizing research methods and concepts from psychology, sociology, administration and policy sciences, economics, and education, program evaluators seek to contribute to the improvement of programs. (p. 2)

Theoretical thinking might be seen as one of the skills, mentioned in this definition, necessary to carry out an effective and program-improving evaluation.

For program evaluators, theory has two important dimensions or two ways in which it becomes relevant: First, theory-driven evaluations consider how theory has been used *within the programs being evaluated* and then use this theory to guide the evaluation plan. Theory-driven evaluators ask questions such as: "*Did the program use behavior change theories to develop its activities?*" "*Which theories were used?*" "*Which theoretical constructs do the programs attempt to influence or change?*" Second, evaluators themselves *think theoretically about their evaluations* and thus reflect theoretically about their practice (asking questions such as these: "*Did my evaluation work?*" "*Did it capture the program's effects, fairly and efficiently?*" "*Which elements of my evaluation yielded the most comprehensive findings?*" "*Was my evaluation of program X fair and just to all stakeholders involved?*"). Both of these theory dimensions tell important stories about programs and about how we assess their impact (Alkin & Christie, 2005). Theoretical thinking about program *evaluations* has been around for a rather long time (at least 30 years, say many evaluators) (Christie, 2003; Donaldson, 2007). Using program theory to *guide* an evaluation, however, became established as a significant practice only in the 1980s and 1990s (despite having been proposed 50 years earlier; see Donaldson, 2007; Henry & Mark, 2003).

Unfortunately, there is "a great deal of confusion today about what is meant by theory-based or theory-driven evaluation," says Stewart Donaldson (2007, p. 9).

The terminology evaluators have employed to refer to this type of evaluation isn't very helpful either, as differences in approaches and methods become obscured by the multitude of labels, including "theory-oriented evaluation, theory-based evaluation, theory-driven evaluation, program theory evaluation, intervening mechanism evaluation, theoretically relevant evaluation research, program theory, program logic, logic modeling" (Donaldson, 2007, p. 9). A rather simple way to understand evaluations that employ theory (social science theories or implicit theories) is this, proposed by Donaldson (2007):

> Simply stated, evaluators typically work with stakeholders to develop a common understanding of how a program is presumed to solve a problem or problems of interest. Social science theory and prior research (if they exist) can be used to inform this discussion, and to assess the feasibility of the proposed relationships between a program and its desired initial, intermediate, and long-term outcomes. . . . This common understanding or program theory helps evaluators and stakeholders identify and prioritize evaluation questions. Evaluation questions of most interest are then answered using the most rigorous scientific methods possible given the practical constraints of the evaluation context. (pp. 10–11)

For the purposes of this book, I focus only on the role of theory as it is used to guide the evaluations. The role of theory in reflecting about and attempting to improve how the *evaluations* (not the programs themselves) are conducted I do not address here. If you are interested in this topic, many of the sources I cite throughout this chapter represent good places to learn about it. I also recommend you familiarize yourself with the American Evaluation Association, a professional organization for evaluators. The organization provides excellent resources for evaluators, including training workshops and conferences (their website address is www.eval.org). Among the many training workshops they offer each year, you will find several focusing on theory-related topics, such as "Advanced Applications of Program Theory," "Theory Driven Evaluation for Assessing and Improving Program Planning, Implementation, and Effectiveness," and "Logic Models as a Platform for Program Evaluation Planning, Implementation, and Use of Findings," among others.

When I reflect on the role theory plays in program evaluation, the first thing that comes to my mind is this: In a sense, almost any program evaluation is itself an exercise in theoretical thinking. If theoretical thinking strives to make sense of reality and if scientific theories focus on causal-type relationships, the central question embedded in most program evaluations is, intrinsically, a theoretical, causal question: "Did the implemented program lead to the desired outcomes?" (Patton, 1997, p. 216), or more specifically, "To what extent and in what ways do the processes, activities, and treatments of a program cause or affect the behaviors, attitudes, skills, knowledge, and feelings of targeted participants?" (Patton, 1997, p. 216). Asking these questions and attempting to answer them are the program evaluator's job. As we learned in Chapter 1, theorizing consists of asking and answering a specific type of question: the questions of "why," "how," or "to what extent." In this sense, program evaluation *is* theoretical thinking at its best.

Yet there are at least two ways in which evaluators can go about asking and answering the "why" or "how" type of questions. One way is to focus on the goal of testing the particular set of theories that guided the program's development and implementation; another way is to focus on the goal of deciphering the kind of impact the program has had upon the problem it tried to address. Let us examine these two ways of focusing an evaluation and what might be the role theory plays in each of them.

APPLYING THEORY TO PROGRAM EVALUATION

Program Evaluation as Theory Testing

Some evaluations seek to test the health promotion theories upon which the programs are based, thus attempting to produce evidence in support (or in denial) of a specific theory. For example, evaluators of a school-based nutrition program may be interested in testing whether Social Cognitive Theory is the most appropriate approach for such a program. Program evaluations that have the purpose of theory testing usually engage in a *deductive* model of evaluation. In other words, these evaluations *begin with the theories* used for grounding the program's outcomes and activities then proceed to collect data and test whether they support or negate the theory within that particular program's context. When this is the case, applying theory to program evaluation becomes akin to applying the guidelines for using theory in a research project (quantitative, qualitative, or mixed methods—see Chapter 8).

Nevertheless, many evaluation scholars are skeptical regarding this deductive, theory-testing perspective and warn us about its potential dangers. Patton (1997), for instance, specifically points out that "the temptation in the deductive approach is to make the study more research than evaluation, that is, to let the literature review and theory testing take over the evaluation" (p. 220).

Patton (1997) adds:

> Theory-driven evaluations can seduce researchers away from answering straight-forward formative questions or determining the merit or worth of a program into the ethereal world of academic theorizing. In this regard, Scriven (1991)

asserts that theory testing is a "luxury for the evaluator." He considers it "a gross though frequent blunder to suppose that one needs a theory of learning to evaluate teaching'" (p. 360). One does not need to know anything at all about electronics, he observes, to evaluate computers. (p. 220)

These warnings are not offered by evaluation scholars who find no value in theory—quite the contrary. These evaluators are theoreticians who ground their own evaluations in solid theory and evidence. Nevertheless, they strongly believe program evaluations should be primarily about generating information that will ultimately be used for program improvement (unfortunately, many evaluation findings are never used to make changes and improvements in programs; see Patton for a thorough and intriguing discussion of this topic). Theory testing can be a "by-product" of program evaluations but should not be their focus; assessing the impact of a program should (Patton, 1997).

Program Evaluation as Assessment of Program Impact

Critics of program evaluation as theory testing don't have much to worry about because *the majority* of evaluations do *not* seek to test a social science or health promotion theory. If most evaluations are not designed to test a given health promotion theory and if an exclusive focus on theory testing betrays the principal functions of program evaluation, can theory play any other relevant role in evaluations?

The answer is "yes!" Even if social science or health promotion theories are not overtly being applied by the program, evaluators can invoke theoretical thinking as an important tool in their evaluation arsenal. *How can they do that?* you ask. *How can theory become a useful tool for evaluators when their main purpose is to learn about the programs and their effectiveness, not to test whether the programs were based on scientific theories, nor if those theories "hold" within the context of that particular program?*

Remember when I discussed earlier in the chapter the importance of developing or identifying a program's implicit theory, internal logic, or theory of action? Remember I also said such a task would prove useful not only for planning the program but also for its future evaluation? Well, *here* is where theory turns out to be tremendously useful once again: Evaluators save themselves a lot of grief if they spend time learning about the program's implicit theory, internal logic, or theory of action. These theories of action (as opposed to general theories of health promotion or behavior change) should be the ones guiding evaluators in their assessment (Patton, 1997, p. 221). These theories specify how to produce results and answer the question, "Why did program X produce (or not) outcome Y?"

Health promotion programs' *theories of action*, then, can serve as valuable guides for evaluators to focus their assessments. According to Donaldson (2007), many are the advantages of using a program's own theoretical framework, in an evaluation: First, it "forces evaluators to try to understand the value and (the program) in some detail before rushing to action" (p. 13); second, it improves the validity and sensitivity of the evaluation plan, allowing evaluators to better capture the "true" effects of the program. If nothing else, focusing on a program's theory of action allows evaluators to identify "pertinent variables and how, when . . . and on whom they should be measured" (Donaldson, 2007, p. 13).

In the earlier portions of this chapter, we examined how one might graph a program's logic, or its theory of action. Ideally, program planners (or program staff) will have developed a model similar to the one in Figure 9–3. Yet, an even more ideal scenario (is there such as thing as "more ideal"?) would be to have had the program evaluators themselves assist program planners in developing the theory of action. As Patton (1997) points out,

> At times, helping program staff or decision makers to articulate their programmatic theory of action is an end in itself. Evaluators are called on, not only to gather data, but also to assist in program design. Knowing how to turn a vague discussion of the presumed linkages between program activities and expected outcomes into a formal written theory of action can be an important service to a program. (p. 229)

But "real world" evaluations rarely engage planners and evaluators, working together, from the inception of the planning process. So, when conducting an evaluation of a program for which you, as the evaluator, did not have a chance to sit at the planning table, you should consider, as one of the first steps in the evaluation, spending some time learning about the program's theory of action (if program staff have developed one). If no program theory is available, you should develop your own, based on information about the program: its activities, immediate, intermediate, and long-term goals. Remember that evaluation of sexual abstinence programs in Texas I mentioned previously? Our evaluation team spent at least 3 months examining the logic models of each program based on their grant proposals. For each one, the team (with the assistance of a group of undergraduate health education students) graphed a logic model, identifying (1) each of the program's planned activities, (2) each activities' inputs, (3) each activities' constraints (and potential barriers), and (4) each activities' expected outcomes. The team also developed a model connecting all program activities to get a better sense of the complexity of the program and how each component related to all others (Borich & Brackett, 1978; Borich & Jemelka, 1982).

This essential first step—identifying, or "uncovering" a program's internal logic—is rather labor intensive and takes time. Remember this when you're planning a program evaluation of your own, but don't be tempted to skip this step because learning about the program's theory of action will help you focus your evaluation, formulate your evaluation questions, and most of all, conduct a fair assessment of the program. One of the models I recommend to help you develop the program's theory of action is presented in the book *Programs and Systems: An Evaluation Perspective*, authored by Gary Borich (once a professor of mine) and Ron Jemelka (1982). This modeling strategy relies on a "structured decomposition" technique, defined by the authors as follows:

> The process of breaking down a program into its component parts. Decomposition begins by graphically dividing the program into a number of general activities, each symbolizing a major class of events within the program. Each general activity is then further broken down into a small number of subactivities in succeeding steps of the process. By introducing substantive detail gradually, and in meaningful steps, a uniform, systematic exposition of successive levels of detail is achieved at the same time that a global conceptualization of the program is maintained. (p. 242)

This tool will only help you unveil a program's theory and understand its basic structure; it won't necessarily guide you through planning an entire evaluation. There are, however, very useful models that can lead you through developing an evaluation design step-by-step. One model used quite extensively in public health is the Centers for Disease Control and Prevention's (CDC) Evaluation Framework (CDC, 1999; Davis, 2006).

The CDC's Evaluation Framework was designed as a "practical, nonprescriptive tool" to help practitioners "summarize and organize the essential elements of program evaluation" (CDC, 1999, p. 8). The framework comprises six steps evaluators must take to implement an effective evaluation, as well as 30 standards (grouped into four categories), proposed as criteria to assess the quality of the evaluation activities themselves. Authors of the framework describe it like this:

> The framework is composed of six steps that must be taken in any evaluation. They are starting points for tailoring an evaluation to a particular public health effort at a particular time. Because the steps are all interdependent, they might be encountered in a nonlinear sequence; however, an order exists for fulfilling each—earlier steps provide the foundation for subsequent progress. Thus, decisions regarding how to execute a step are iterative and should not be finalized until previous steps have been thoroughly addressed. The steps are as follows:
>
> Step 1: Engage stakeholders
> Step 2: Describe the program

Step 3: Focus the evaluation design
Step 4: Gather credible evidence
Step 5: Justify conclusions
Step 6: Ensure use and share lessons learned

. . . The second element of the framework is a set of 30 standards for assessing the quality of evaluation activities, organized into the following four groups:

Standard 1: utility . . . are information needs of evaluation users satisfied?
Standard 2: feasibility . . . is the evaluation viable and pragmatic?
Standard 3: propriety . . . is the evaluation ethical?
Standard 4: accuracy . . . are the evaluation findings correct?

These standards . . . answer the question, "Will this evaluation be effective?" and are recommended as criteria for judging the quality of program evaluation efforts in public health. (CDC, 1999, pp. 8–9, 20)

If one examines this framework closely, it is not difficult to perceive that theory can play an especially useful role in Step 2: Describing the Program. As we have seen, one way in which programs can be described, is by breaking the down the program into its main components (the programs' activities or tasks) and to uncover the logic connecting the activities to the desired outcome (remember the question my research team had to ask of certain abstinence programs: "*How does dancing lead to abstinence?*"—which I described in Chapter 3?). Unveiling a program's implicit theory becomes therefore an essential "piece" of this evaluation framework.

The authors of the CDC framework (1999) call this process of uncovering a program's theory of action, developing a "Logic Model":

A logic model describes the sequence of events for bringing about change by synthesizing the main program elements into a picture of how the program is supposed to work. Often, this model is displayed in a flow chart, map, or table to portray the sequence of steps leading to program results. . . . One of the virtues of a logic model is its ability to summarize the program's overall mechanism of change by linking processes (e.g., laboratory diagnosis of disease) to eventual effects (e.g., reduced tuberculosis incidence). . . . A detailed logic model can also strengthen claims of causality [theory] and be a basis for estimating the program's effect on endpoints that are not directly measured but are linked in a causal chain supported by prior research. (p. 11)

Yet, not only is theory useful in Step 2 of the CDC's Evaluation Framework to facilitate the process of describing a program's internal logic: Theorizing is the core element when it comes to applying the evaluation standards. Think about it: When evaluators stop and ask specific questions about their evaluation (*Is it accurate? Is it ethical?*), the act of asking and answering these questions—as we discussed earlier in this book—*is* theoretical thinking. Such theorizing may not come associated with scientific or behavior change theories, but it *is* theoretical thinking nonetheless—perhaps even *theoretical thinking at its best!*

SUGGESTIONS FOR PRACTICING THEORETICAL THINKING

1. Plan and hold a panel discussion with colleagues involved in developing and evaluating different programs in public health. Ask the panelists to tell their stories of how theory was used (or not) in the planning and evaluation activities in which they participated.
2. Reflect on the distinction between "ideal" and "real-world" strategies for applying theory into program planning. Does this distinction match your experience? If it does, can you think of specific examples?
3. Become familiar (if you are not, yet) with the PRECEDE–PROCEED model and with Intervention Mapping. Explore their discussions about incorporating theory into planning, implementing and evaluating health promotion programs.
4. Practice graphing or outlining a program's implicit theory. You can do this exercise by choosing a program for which several evaluation reports have been published (e.g., the CATCH program, or Coordinated Approach to Child Health, available from http://www.catchinfo.org). Practice developing a theory-of-action model based on the information these publications provide about the program.
5. Based on the model you developed in number 4, see whether you can generate a set of evaluation questions. Ask yourself: Will answering these questions provide data to test the program's internal logic or theory of action?

REFERENCES

Alkin, M. C., & Christie, C. A. (Eds.). (2005). *Theorists' Models in Action*. San Francisco: Jossey-Bass and the American Evaluation Association.

Bartholomew, L. K., Parcel, G. S., Kok, G., & Gottlieb, N. H. (2006). *Planning Health Promotion Programs: An Intervention Mapping Approach*. 2nd ed. San Francisco, Jossey-Bass.

Borich, G. D., & Brackett, J. W. (1978). Instructional program design and evaluation with a structured analysis and design technique. *Educational Technology, 18*(7), 18–23.

Borich, G. D., & Jemelka, R. P. (1982). *Programs and Systems: An Evaluation Perspective*. New York: Academic Press.

Centers for Disease Control and Prevention. (1999). Framework for program evaluation in public health. *Morbidity and Mortality Weekly Report (MMWR), 48*(No. RR-11), (inclusive page numbers).

Champion, V. L., & Skinner, C. S. (2008). The health belief model. In K. Glanz, B. K. Rimer, & K. Viswanath (Eds.), *Health Behavior and Health Education: Theory, Research, and Practice*. (4th ed., pp. 45–65). San Francisco: Jossey-Bass.

Christie, C. A. (2003). What guides evaluation? A study of how evaluation practice maps onto evaluation theory. In C. A. Christie (Ed.), *The Practice-Theory Relationship in Evaluation* (pp. 7–35). San Francisco: Jossey-Bass.

Davis, M. V. (2006). Teaching practical public health evaluation methods. *American Journal of Evaluation, 27*(2), 247–256.

Donaldson, S. I. (2007). *Program Theory-Driven Evaluation Science: Strategies and Applications*. New York: Lawrence Erlbaum Associates.

Gielen, A. C., McDonald, E. M., Gary, T. L., & Bone, L. R. (2008). Using the Precede-Proceed model to apply health behavior theories. In K. Glanz, B. K. Rimer, & K. Viswanath (Eds.), *Health Behavior and Health Education: Theory, Research, and Practice* (pp. 407–433). San Francisco: Jossey-Bass.

Goodson, P., Pruitt, B. E., Suther, S., Wilson, K., & Buhi, E. (2006). Is abstinence education theory based? The underlying logic of abstinence education programs in Texas. *Health Education & Behavior, 33*(2), 252–271.

Green, L. W., & Kreuter, M. W. (2005). *Health Program Planning: An Educational and Ecological Approach* (4th ed.). Boston: McGraw-Hill.

Henry, G. T., & Mark, M. M. (2003). Toward an agenda for research on evaluation. In C. A. Christie (Ed.), *The Practice-Theory Relationship in Evaluation* (pp. 69–80). San Francisco: Jossey-Bass.

Hochbaum, G. M., Sorenson, J. R., & Lorig, K. (1992). Theory in health education practice. *Health Education Quarterly, 19*(3), 295–313.

Lewin, K. (1951). *Field Theory in Social Science: Selected Theoretical Papers*. New York: Harper & Brothers Publishers.

McQueen, D. V., Kickbusch, I., Potvin, L., Pelikan, J. M., Balbo, L., & Abel, T. (2007). *Health and Modernity: The Role of Theory in Health Promotion*. New York: Springer.

Patton, M. Q. (1997). *Utilization-Focused Evaluation: The New Century Text*. Thousand Oaks, CA: Sage Publications.

Posavac, E. J., & Carey, R. G. (2007). *Program Evaluation: Methods and Case Studies* (7th ed.). Upper Saddle River, NJ: Pearson/Prentice Hall.

Scriven, M. (1991). *Evaluation Thesaurus* (4th ed.). Newbury Park, CA: Sage Publications.

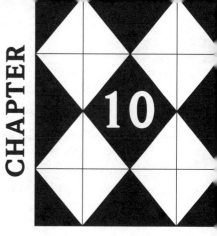

CHAPTER 10

Bridging the Gap: Recommendations to Enhance the Use of Theory in Health Promotion Research and Practice

Learning Objectives

When you finish reading this chapter, you will be able to:

1. Point to specific strategies for strengthening the theory–practice relationship in health promotion.
2. Explain why theorizing in health promotion should move beyond the goal of predicting and changing health behaviors to questioning its purpose and meaning.

3. Describe how your training program incorporates and teaches (or incorporated and presented, if you have already graduated) health promotion theories.

4. List a few options for changing the way in which health promotion theories are taught in many public health training programs.

5. Ask the "hard question": Where is the "education" in health education efforts?

6. Consider ways in which you might begin to think theoretically "outside the box" in your field.

THIS FAR . . .

If you read this book in sequence, you will recall that in the previous chapters I defined theories as stories that are told to make sense of reality. I also distinguished between commonsense and scientific theories, pointing to their unique characteristics and to their shared feature: Both types of theories tell stories about human realities related to health and illness, well-being, and dis-*ease*. I pointed out, emphatically, that theory *is* a form of practice, that theory (or more precisely theoretical thinking) *does* several important things: It attributes meaning to human realities; it asks and answers specific types of questions; it questions the status quo and builds a narrative or logical structure for the questions and the answers.

In Chapters 4 through 7, you journeyed through the current "theoretical landscape" in public health and examined several of its blind spots. Finally, in the last two chapters, I offered specific guidelines for choosing and applying theory to research, program planning, and evaluation efforts.

There remains, however, one more stop in the journey—one last point to consider. We cannot declare the journey complete without considering possible strategies for solving the theoretical "conundrum" that public health faces. The strategies I offer here are not my original ideas, and they have been proposed before by other theoretical thinkers in the field. Nevertheless, because I urged you throughout this text to think theoretically *about* health promotion, I would like to put forth one final challenge: that of developing better solutions for bridging the theory–practice divide that seems so relentless and so ubiquitous in our field. So, for a moment, let us consider this question: What can be done in health promotion/public health to enhance the development and application of theoretical thinking so both the profession and society at large may benefit?"

FRAMING THE GAP

In Chapter 3 you read about three different paradigms commonly used to explain or to "frame" the relationship between theory and practice. The first paradigm postulates the relationship between theory and practice as one of diffusion and utilization of knowledge (knowledge moves in the direction of theory *to* practice exclusively); the second paradigm offers a political perspective to the relationship, affirming the association between theory and practice is determined ultimately by the political and economic forces that affect scientists and practitioners, and the third paradigm proposes theory and practice interact much in the same way two distinct cultural groups might relate to each other: through an acculturation, or reciprocal influence process.

Invariably, any recommendation made by researchers and practitioners regarding how to "bridge the gap" between theory/research and practice is a by-product of the paradigm employed to understand the relationship in the first place. Those that perceive the relationship between academics and practitioners (theory and practice) as one of knowledge diffusion will recommend a better understanding of the Diffusion of Innovations Theory itself. Examining the theory helps diagnose which elements of the dissemination and communication processes can be changed to enhance the use of theory or the application of scientific knowledge into practice (Dearing, 2004; Sobell, 1996). Dearing, for instance, suggests that a clearer understanding of the factors involved in diffusing knowledge from academic circles to the field will accelerate the dissemination process while simultaneously making it more efficient.

Similarly, for those who see the relationship between theory and practice as one determined mainly by political ideologies and economic systems, enhancing the relationship between theory and practice must happen at the level of community, state, and federal politics and policies. Scientists and practitioners alike must involve themselves in their political systems and attempt to influence the "powers that be" in order that research, intervention, and evaluation funding may eventually converge and lead to a better relationship between the academy and the field. In other words, researchers and practitioners need to look "outside" their work environments for potential solutions to enhancing their interactions.

An example of this interplay between public health and political systems was the U.S. Congress enacting legislation to authorize the creation of Health Promotion and Disease Prevention Research Centers (PRC) nationwide in 1984 (Riley & Kaplan, 1999). Viewed as a "network of academic centers for prevention research" (p. 5), proponents of this initiative

... convinced Congress of the importance of supporting a public health research program that could directly affect public health practice. . . . the program's proponents were resolute in their belief that [the] PRC program was the vehicle that could bridge academic research and community practice in a way that had not yet occurred. (p. 5)

Finally, those who propose scientists and practitioners inhabit different "cultures" believe the relationship between the two *can* improve, but significant cultural obstacles must be overcome. Cross (1999), for instance, affirms,

> Successful collaboration between academia and practice requires bridging this gap between the two *cultures, their values, and their priorities.* The best way to understand a different culture is to take time to live in the foreign environment and allow yourself to be subject to its varied norms, rules, and subtleties. To foster better collaborations we need more opportunities for practitioners to spend time in the academy and for academics to work in practice settings. Those who have such experiences can also serve as cultural translators for others. . . . . True linkages will be forged only when there are enough people on each side who understand and respect the realities of the other side. (p. 14, emphasis mine)

I provided a summary of these paradigms for understanding the relationship between theory and practice in Table 3–1 in Chapter 3. That table does not, however, account for the fact that in reality many health promotion scholars embrace a comprehensive view of the theory–practice relationship and, when making recommendations for bridging the divide, will often mention elements from all of the paradigms described in the table. A case in point is Morrissey and colleagues (1997). In a study entitled, "*Toward a Framework for Bridging the Gap Between Science and Practice in Prevention: A Focus on Evaluator and Practitioner Perspectives,*" the authors list a series of recommendations for minimizing the distance between prevention science and practice. Within this list, many of the suggestions directly reflect one or more of the three main paradigms described previously (for more detail, see Chapter 3). For instance (Morrissey et al., 1997)

- Seek and disseminate information from prevention research scientists to prevention practitioners (recommendation made for program evaluators based on the diffusion model).
- Train prevention practitioners to access the prevention science literature (recommendation made for program evaluators based on the diffusion model).
- Work in communities to serve as translators of scientific constructs (recommendation made for research scientists based on the acculturation model).

- Increase funding for technical transfer of prevention science and for improving the technology of technical transfer between the science and practice sectors (recommendation for regional and national prevention agencies based on the political perspective model). (p. 375)

Another useful example of how recommendations for bridging the gap between theory and practice can contain elements from all three paradigms is the four-gap model proposed by Lancaster in 1992. The four main gaps he identified as problematic for health promotion theory and practice were the communications gap, accessibility gap, credibility gap, and expectations gap. In 2000, Lancaster and Roe reexamined health education's efforts in the past decade to address these gaps. Their examination, published in an article in *Health Promotion Practice*, concluded (Lancaster & Roe, 2000):

> The decade of the 1990s may eventually be known as the decade of closing the gaps between practice and research in health education and health promotion. Newer ecological theories and models . . . , healthy cities and communities movements . . . , participatory action research . . . , empowerment evaluation . . . , and community capacity and social capital . . . are areas of increased interest that lend themselves to links between researchers and practitioners as well as with community groups. (pp. 35–36)

But viewing the theory–practice and researcher–practitioner relationship comprehensively, or in a manner that incorporates elements from the various models we described, is not the same as embracing a *theory-as-practice*, or *dialogical model* (described in Chapter 1) for understanding the relationship. If we embrace the point of view that theory *is* practice, that the relationship between theory and practice is dynamic, synergistic, and holistic, then the question we should be asking is "How can the theory-practice relationship be *strengthened*?" instead of asking how it can be *bridged. How can the integration and the "oneness" of theory and practice be sustained more effectively? Is it enough to follow the recommendations found in each of the paradigms examined here, or should a more outside-the-box approach be implemented?*

I would like to propose—in addition to the recommendations offered by scholars in each of the three paradigms described previously—a few strategies that I believe hold the key to important changes in the way we think about theory and practice. These strategies are: Shifting the process of theory building in health promotion, changing health promoters' professional training regarding theory, adapting the processes of knowledge building (or research) in health promotion, and taking a hard look at our health promotion practice as a whole (Buchanan, 2000). As I said previously, I did not create these strategies—I have borrowed heavily, once again, from David Buchanan, as he represents one of the main proponents of a radical shift in the theorizing process in health promotion. Let's examine then each of these tactics more closely.

STRATEGIES TO BRIDGE THE GAP

Shifting the Process of Theory Building in Health Promotion

For Buchanan, health promotion theories should move *beyond explaining* human behavior as a means to its prediction and control. Theories should seek to clarify assumptions underlying human actions and understand the aims, intentions, purposes, and meanings of behaviors (Buchanan, 1994, 1998, 2000). These processes (of clarifying and understanding) cannot be carried out unilaterally and presuppose both that (1) collaboration between practitioners and researchers is needed to develop this sort of theory and (2) that such types of theories meet practitioners' needs at many more levels than current theories do (Buchanan, 1998).

In his book *An Ethic for Health Promotion* (2000), Buchanan provides carefully crafted and very compelling arguments for the need to shift the process of theory building in health promotion (for a more in-depth look at Buchanan's arguments, I refer the reader to that book, as well as to some of his journal articles listed in this chapter's reference section). In these pieces, he contrasts the *scientific model* of health promotion and its use of theory with a *humanistic model* (or a *practical reasoning model*) and its use of theory (see Figure 10–1 for an illustration of both models I created based on Buchanan's arguments).

In the scientific model, theory refers to a set of statements from which hypotheses can be derived. After these hypotheses are stated, they can be tested empirically with data. Developing and testing these hypotheses lead to the identification of a set of factors (or determinants) that *cause* a phenomenon of interest. If the causes of a phenomenon are known, the phenomenon itself can be manipulated, changed, modified.

As an example, consider childhood obesity as a phenomenon of interest. Health behavior theories that try to explain the causes of childhood obesity are numerous; many of them propose that parents model eating behavior in the home. Whether parents influence their children's eating by modeling specific eating behaviors becomes, therefore, a hypothesis that can be generated by these health behavior theories. If, after data collection and extensive testing, researchers

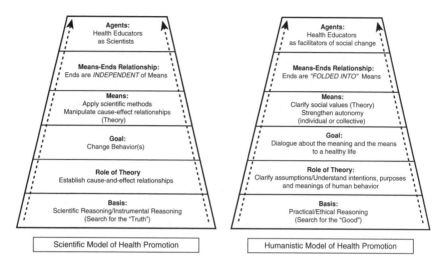

FIGURE 10–1 Two Models of Health Promotion (adapted from Buchanan, 2006)

come to the conclusion that yes, parents do model eating behaviors for their children and this modeling may cause (or prevent) childhood obesity, health promoters can then do something about the problem: They can develop health education programs focusing on parents' eating behaviors and the manner in which those behaviors are modeled in the home. The program can, therefore, expect to change parents' modeling behaviors and, consequently, affect children's eating habits and obesity levels.

In summary, within the scientific model, theory leads researchers to finding the *causes* of human behaviors and subsequently the ways to "*cure*" those behaviors that are problematic (Buchanan, 2004). But health promoters must ask the hard question: Has the scientific model of theorizing been "working"? Have health behavior theories proven to be powerful enough to predict and control the causes of a given health behavior (for instance, children's eating)? Are health promoters increasingly more effective in preventing or changing those factors that lead to childhood obesity (to keep with our previous example)? Buchanan (2004), for instance, sees no evidence of this:

> If we had even only modestly successful theories about what causes people to eat too much, for example, then according to the standards of the scientific model, we would know this by the fact that we could consistently predict and control at least minimal changes in the dependent variable, weight loss. But I do not

think that anyone can seriously contend that weight loss programs are becoming more effective or that we can reliably change any other human behavior, such as making people exercise more, preventing smoking, or eliminating elicit drug use. (p. 149)

Buchanan and other scholars (such as Blumer, 1970) propose that given the apparent ineffectiveness of the scientific model of theorizing, a humanistic (or practical reasoning) model might yield more ethical and meaningful health promotion "results." In Buchanan's (2004) own words,

> In the humanistic model, researchers put forward theories not for the purpose of testing hypothesis but for striving to articulate and *provide greater clarity about the societal values* embodied in different social practices and different institutional arrangements.
> *When theory is so defined, then the relationship between theory and practice is transformed.* Practitioners use theory to stimulate dialogue, seeking to reach reasoned mutual agreement about ways of living that we find most worthwhile. (p. 152, emphasis mine)

Ironically, my study of human sexuality practitioners and researchers (described in Chapter 3) is probably the only "bit" of empirical evidence available on this topic (Goodson & Cheatham, 2002). I asked a sample of members of two large professional organizations dealing with human sexuality (see Chapter 3) whether they believed theories could be more useful if they underwent the transformation Buchanan proposes and began to focus more on the *meanings* of human behaviors rather than on their *causes*. In that study, most researchers and practitioners agreed that theories would be more useful if they focused on the meanings and goals of human behavior, instead of merely on its *causes*.

Despite generalized agreement that a change in theorizing could benefit the field, can such a shift actually happen? As we see in later sections, this shift requires many other, concomitant changes: changes in the value we place upon empirical/scientifically developed knowledge as the only valid way of knowing the truth about (or causes of) a phenomenon, changes in the methods we would use to acquire other types of knowledge judged to be as valuable as scientific knowledge; changes in how researchers and practitioners practice their professional callings and careers. Whether these changes will be implemented in public health and health promotion training programs remains to be seen. Rethinking the relationship between theory and practice and viewing the relationship as a dynamic, synergistic unity, however, represents an important first step.

Changing Health Promoters' Professional Training Regarding Theory

Whether operating from a scientific model of theorizing or from a humanistic model, academic training programs in health promotion, health education, and public health would do well to examine the beliefs regarding the theory–practice and researcher–practitioner relationships that their curricula overtly (or covertly) promote. Which model (or paradigm) of the relationship between theory and practice is being taught and modeled throughout the curricula? Are theory and practice perceived as dichotomous and polarized? Are practitioners viewed as passive consumers of theoretical knowledge, or are they portrayed as active subjects in the knowledge development process? Is theory being taught exclusively in a health–behavior theories course, or is it being integrated continually within courses such as program planning and evaluation? Are students being encouraged to memorize constructs from selected theories, or are they being taught the logical and critical thinking skills associated with theoretical thinking and with applying theory to research and practice? Are students being led to think critically or to reflect theoretically (and, therefore, ethically) about their practice?

Alongside examining the beliefs and assumptions about theory and practice being communicated, programs should also assess whether their training proactively fosters students' mastery of the integration of theory and practice. Hochbaum, Sorenson, and Lorig (1992) believe, for instance, that "the underutilization of theories in health education practice is due less to an oversupply of theories and more to inadequate training in *using* them" (p. 311). While systematically collected data are not available on this topic, my interactions with faculty and students in health promotion programs nationwide reveal that health behavior theory courses focus—for the most part—on two major elements: descriptions of the numerous theories used in health promotion practice and research (on the part of the instructors) and memorization of these theories' main constructs and characteristics on the part of the students. Application of theory into practice is either neglected due to time limitations or hastily added as an afterthought (Hochbaum et al., 1992).

Changes in health promotion training regarding the integration of theory and practice would entail a close partnership between academia and the field to allow health promotion students "real-live" opportunities to infuse practice with theory and to connect their theoretical thinking to action. Several models to promote the merging of classroom and community-based experiences have been proposed (see D'Onofrio, 1992; Helitzer & Wallerstein, 1999; Institute of Medicine, 1988).

Perhaps more systematic application of some of these curriculum models could contribute significantly to narrowing the gap between theory and practice.

In tandem with the proposition to shift the theorizing process in health promotion, Buchanan (2000) also proposed changes to the health promotion curriculum. He suggested, for instance, that the curriculum "could be improved by incorporating historical investigations" (p. 146). Adding a historical perspective and history-related theories to health promotion curricula is essential for improved understanding of the issues we face in the field today. In Buchanan's (2000) words,

> The history of health promotion is replete with the rise and fall of periodic health crusades, proud accomplishments and quirky fads. Entering professionals would be well served by reviewing this history, thereby gaining a critical perspective on current trends and their own motives for entering the field. (p. 146)

Another change Buchanan recommends is a greater focus on the ethical foundations of our field. Come to think of it, when was the last time you—as a student—enrolled in an Ethics of Health Promotion class? There is a strong probability that even if you had wished to sit in such a class the course was not offered at your institution. If you were fortunate enough to have had such a course in your curriculum, I would venture to say that its focus was mainly on ethical concerns of the field or what has been technically named "bioethics" (Buchanan, 2000). A covert focus on the ethical foundations of health promotion, nevertheless, would require a slightly different approach from the one subsumed in bioethics courses. A stronger focus on moral philosophy and theory-assessment skills would be needed in order to foster students' critical analysis of the field's main assumptions, beliefs, and practices.

A final change in the health promotion training curriculum would involve teaching and learning other research methods and approaches to knowledge building (Buchanan, 2000; Hochbaum et al., 1992). Because to shift epistemologies is not a small task, it deserves to be examined as a category all its own, and therefore, I describe these alternative research methods and approaches later. Nevertheless, I mention this change here because it would become a shift that would also affect our curricula and training.

Adapting the Processes of Knowledge Building (or Research) in Health Promotion

Hand in hand with the proposal to shift the process of theorizing in health promotion, the need for broader utilization of naturalistic-type approaches to research (see a description of this approach in Chapter 8) has been advocated by several scholars (Green & Mercer, 2001; Israel, Schulz, Parker, & Becker, 1998; Minkler, 2000). Although the scientific model in health promotion may be useful for answering specific types of questions, the *ethical foundations of such a model may be inconsistent with the mission of health promotion*, especially when it comes to understanding and helping to foster voluntary behavior changes. Does it make sense for health promoters to operate within a paradigm that claims to be "value free," all the while having, as its main goal, the promotion of something health researchers value intensely (health)? Is it reasonable or even ethical to approach community-based research of health-related issues with a posture that claims complete distance and disengagement between researcher and the "object" of the research? Can health promotion research and practice be completely "aseptic" and void of assumptions, perspectives, social and cultural norms, as well as personal norms (Lincoln & Guba, 1985)? Not only should we consider whether health promotion research can fit the "clean" scientific model, but we also should ask ourselves whether it *should* be made to fit such model.

Precisely because the scientific model of knowledge building—in terms of its own internal ethical system—may actually be at odds with the ethical principles guiding the practice of health promotion, other models must be examined and tested for their suitability. One such model that deserves strong consideration as an alternative to the scientific-positivistic one is participatory action research (or PAR—also known as Community-Based Participatory Action Research, or CBPAR). As defined by Green and Mercer (2001), participatory research "is an approach that entails involving all potential users of the research and other stakeholders in the formulation as well as the application of the research" (p. 1927). PAR can be broadly described as research that embodies the following characteristics (Schwandt, 2001):

1. *Is participatory in character*—the researchers collaborate with research participants to define the research question(s) (or problem), the methods for data collection and analysis, and how findings will be utilized;
2. *Has a "democratic impulse"*—in other words, incorporates principles, ideas, and practices that are democratic in nature;
3. *Is oriented toward producing both useful knowledge and action as well as consciousness raising.* (p. 187)

In summary, participatory action research provides opportunities for nonresearchers and for those affected directly by the research enterprise to provide input to examine and test assumptions being made by scientists and to pilot-test practice (Minkler, 2000). According to Green and Mercer (2001), "participatory research—research that is generated collaboratively in a partnership between scientists and others—has reemerged in recent decades as an alternative to top-down technical assistance from experts to practitioners or community residents . . ." (p. 1926).

Another approach to research that would prove useful for health promotion knowledge building is the qualitative, case-study approach. Buchanan (2000), for instance, specifically proposes that health promotion courses be *built around* qualitative case studies in order to allow students the opportunity to practice theoretical–critical reflection regarding the research development process:

> Rather than learning sets of variables from select theories of human behavior to be used in defining operational program objectives, students need intensive practice in examining morally complex situations in order to apprehend more clearly the good and bad parts in actual community programs. (p. 146)

He also points out that organizing course work around particular case studies is not a new pedagogical strategy, having been used very successfully in medicine, business, marketing, and law schools (Buchanan, 2000).

Taking a Hard Look at Health Promotion Practice

Unless we as health promotion professionals are willing to ask some theoretically "hard" questions of our own practice and are willing to use theory in its most useful aspect—that of questioning the status quo (Nealon & Giroux, 2003)—unless we are willing to ask of ourselves

- *What* have we been doing?
- *How* have we been practicing our profession?
- *Where* are we headed with our current ways of practice?
- *When* have we been effective?

the "gap" between theory and practice will remain untouched and perhaps even continue to widen. We should not become complacent and assume that "business as usual" in our field is harmless.

We must always keep in mind that health promotion, since its beginnings, has suffered from a protracted case of identity crisis. Public health (health promotion and health education specifically) has always wanted to look more like science. In order to appear more scientific, public health has had to focus on phenomena that can be observed, measured, and captured through a researcher's five physical senses. Only *these* factors can legitimately be studied, understood, and manipulated, says science. In the case of human health, in order to become aligned with the scientific method, we observe unhealthy behaviors (applying biological or psychological measures), break them down into their smaller parts (attitudes, beliefs, and social pressures), find which element is most likely causing the behaviors (e.g., the person's beliefs), develop and implement an intervention to affect those beliefs, and *voila!* The unhealthy behaviors disappear; in their place, a new set of healthy practices. By focusing on behaviors and how to change them, health promotion found potentially promising solutions for its identity crisis: (1) It could help people adopt healthy behaviors more quickly and readily than if it focused on changing political structures to promote health, and (2) it made health promotion look more like science, gaining in political status and thus appearing more legitimate.

Such focus on changing behaviors might have allowed health promotion to become more science-like, but it ignored one very important reality: Health behaviors, health promotion, and the ways in which people manage their *diseased* conditions are not matters that can be fully handled by science. All of these elements may contain a few bits and pieces that can be *informed* by the scientific method, but because they are human behaviors and because humans are much more than their genetic makeup, their bodies, and even their brains, human behavior—especially health behaviors—has significant moral, political, and spiritual components. Science is not the appropriate lens for examining these components. It is far too limited.

Inevitably, this imposition of a scientific agenda on a field dealing largely with nonscientifically determined matters has created multiple tensions for health promotion specifically and for the field of public health as a whole. One important tension has been the absence of marked effectiveness of health promotion programs. Buchanan (2000) somberly reminds us

> A growing mass of evidence shows that the most carefully designed scientific interventions intended to reduce modern health problems have not proven successful. Carefully controlled, scientifically designed health promotion interventions—such as the many heart disease prevention programs (the Stanford three- and five-community studies, the Minnesota Heart Health plan, the Pawtucket trials, the Karelia intervention), the highly intensive and individualized Multiple Risk Factor Intervention Trials (MRFIT), and the more recent National Cancer Institute (NCI)-sponsored smoking reduction plan, the Community Intervention Trial (COMMIT)—have produced little evidence of success. In reviewing the results of these many large scale randomized control trials, even ardent advocates of the science of health promotion acknowledge that they have produced "disappointing results." (p. 10)

Another tension (almost a contradiction) can be found in the label "health education" itself (Buchanan, 2000). The tension stems from each of the terms reflecting an entirely different paradigm for health promotion. The word "health" currently points to a medical model of health behavior and health promotion; the label "education" suggests a humanistic model. Both models, according to Buchanan, offer "interesting contrasting characteristics" (p. 290).

As public health professionals, we've become familiar with the medical or scientific model for health promotion, but where do we find the *educational* model? One couldn't tell that "education" is a critical element of health promotion by examining the theories I listed in Table 4–1 (in Chapter 4). The list contains only three theories that might loosely be considered "educational" theories: Social Cognitive Theory, Communications Theory, and Freire's Model of Adult Education (this one at least has the word "education" in the title). The absence of educational/learning theories is pronounced, especially when one considers the large number of such theories in existence. If you check out the Theory Into Practice Database on the Internet, for instance, you will find "descriptions of over 50 theories relevant to human learning and instruction" (Kearsley, 1994).

Asking where is the "education" in health education/health promotion most certainly represents one of the hard questions we must direct at our professional field. Not only are theories of teaching and learning conspicuously absent from the current theoretical arsenal, also missing is a philosophy or an approach, a paradigm, for thinking about health promotion in educational terms. In fact, specific theories of human learning are missing, precisely because there is an absence of an educational approach, or paradigm. Here's what Buchanan (2000) proposes we seriously consider regarding a humanistic/educational model for health promotion:

> There are, of course, many different ideas about the purposes of education, so let me start by saying that the model that I have in mind is neither simple information transmission nor vocational skills training (such as auto mechanic school). It is, instead, the model of a broad liberal arts education, where the goal is to develop a cultivated "well-educated" mind. Five common purposes of a liberal education cited in the literature are (a) to enhance one's faculty of critical judgment; (b) to gain deeper self-understanding; (c) to liberate, or free people from narrow, distorted, or prejudiced views of the world; (d) to refine moral sensibilities, by challenging and strengthening one's convictions and sense of obligation to advance justice in this world; and (e) to build respect for the diversity of understandings of the good life for human beings and a commitment to reaching reasoned agreement about how we can best share a more decent and humane world. . . . These purposes, I think, provide a better analogy for thinking about aims of health education. It is exactly what we do, in our best moments, as faculty members and graduate students. (p. 296)

Buchanan further develops each of these five characteristics in his article, and I do encourage you to read it in the near future. Essentially, what is needed is for the next generation of public health professionals (and I'm thinking specifically of health educators here) to consider aligning health education more closely with an educational model, seeking to foster the goals of liberal education among the general public. Instead of focusing exclusively on techniques for changing people's behavior, we should concentrate on increasing human autonomy, enhancing people's critical judgment abilities, fostering self-understanding and self-awareness, refining moral sensibilities, and promoting respect for diverse thinking—all of which are the goals of an educational model, based on principles of ethics and social justice. None of these goals can be achieved through scientific methods. None.

It is imperative, therefore, that we take time to reflect and to ask many hard questions of our profession. Alongside the questions we addressed previously (*Where is the "education" in health education theories?*), we should also reflect on similar questions, such as:

- To what extent are we neglecting to uncover and to question the basic assumptions that underlie the development of knowledge and the delivery of services in public health?
- What has been the main goal of academic teaching of theories—to predict, change, and eventually manipulate people's behavior exclusively?
- Are the means being used to understand health behaviors (behavioral theories and scientific research) the only appropriate means to promote them?
- Should students' mastery to employ health behavioral theories with the purpose of controlling and changing unhealthy behaviors be, in fact, promoted?
- Is theory being used to question the practice of health promotion at all?

Perhaps in raising these questions and their answers, practitioners and scientists could come together to reflect on the need for reforming current academic training and field practice, with the goal of better outcomes for both. Findings from my study of practitioners and researchers in the field of sexual health (described in Chapter 3) indicated that many of those professionals were indeed ready to participate in this process of reflection over assumptions, means, and goals of sexual health research and practice. I would dare to predict that professionals in other areas of health promotion are equally ready to engage in such reflection. I certainly hope *you* are.

FINAL THOUGHTS

As we come to the end of this book, it is my sincere wish for you that you have been challenged to think about theory and its uses in public health research and practice in new, outside-the-box ways.

I am the first to acknowledge that thinking outside the box generally creates tension and quite often frustration because not everyone is ready to reflect on their professional practice in ways that might feel threatening, complex, or challenging. Yet, it is my strong belief that change happens only through tensions and contradictions; through repeated disappointing attempts of doing "business as usual" and obtaining the same, unsatisfying results (what is that definition of insanity, again? *Doing the same thing over and over, expecting a different result each time?*).

It is not difficult to find evidence that public health has, in fact, been quite successful over time; yet, it's easy to see that most of public health's successes have stemmed from changes in environmental conditions, or in policies and laws. The outcomes from behavioral-type interventions, as Buchanan said, remain "disappointing" at best. Isn't it time we think theoretically about *why* this might be the case? Don't we have the moral obligation to admit limited success and attempt to uncover new approaches, new perspectives?

It was my goal, in this chapter and in this book as a whole to challenge you, to push you toward embracing the hard questions, making them your own, and letting go of the fear to ask them. As you accept the challenge, just remember that theoretical thinking comprises both *asking* and *answering*, therefore, it's time you begin to seek out some answers or develop your own. Now, go and think outside the box!

SUGGESTIONS FOR PRACTICING THEORETICAL THINKING

1. Talk to your colleagues; ask about their experiences with learning about theory in their health promotion training. Identify the positive aspects of these experiences; point out the negative ones and how they could be improved.

2. Examine a sample of scientific studies published in your area of interest: How are these studies using theory? Do the authors explicitly mention a health promotion theory? Do they present and explain the theoretical constructs being examined in the study? Do they provide logical explanations of any kind, linking the variables being measured in the study? In summary, what is the "status" of theory-use in your area of expertise?

3. Identify in your training program courses or seminars in which the process of shifting theory building could be started or employed. Are there "places" in your academic program that would benefit from examinations of historical aspects of the profession? Does your program have an ethics of health promotion course, or are ethical issues embedded throughout several courses in the curriculum? Discuss these issues with your colleagues and professors who might be open to following some of the recommendations I put forth in this chapter.

REFERENCES

Blumer, H. (1970). What is wrong with social theory? In N. Denzin (Ed.), *Sociological Methods: A Sourcebook* (pp. 23–45). Chicago: Aldine Publishing Company.

Buchanan, D. R. (1994). Reflections on the relationship between theory and practice. *Health Education Research: Theory & Practice, 9*(3), 273–283.

Buchanan, D. R. (1998). Beyond positivism: humanistic perspectives on theory and research in health education. *Health Education Research: Theory & Practice, 13*(3), 439–450.

Buchanan, D. R. (2000). *An Ethic for Health Promotion: Rethinking the Sources of Human Well-Being*. New York: Oxford University Press.

Buchanan, D. R. (2004). Two models for defining the relationship between theory and practice in nutrition education: is the scientific method meeting our needs? *Journal of Nutrition Education and Behavior, 36,* 146–154.

Cross, A. W. (1999). Bridging the gap between academia and practice in public health. *American Journal of Preventive Medicine, 16*(3S), 14–15.

D'Onofrio, C. N. (1992). Theory and the empowerment of health education practitioners. *Health Education Quarterly, 19,* 385–403.

Dearing, J. W. (2004). Improving the state of health programming by using Diffusion Theory. *Journal of Health Communication, 9,* 21–36.

Goodson, P., & Cheatham, C. (2002). *Beliefs, Self-Efficacy and Barriers Affecting the Integration of Theory, Research and Practice: A Survey of Human Sexuality Academics and Practitioners*. College Station, TX: Texas A&M University, Department of Health & Kinesiology.

Green, L. W., & Mercer, S. L. (2001). Can Public Health researchers and agencies reconcile the push from funding bodies and the pull from communities? *American Journal of Public Health, 91,* 1926–1929.

Helitzer, D., & Wallerstein, N. (1999). A proposal for a graduate curriculum integrating theory and practice in public health. *Health Education Research: Theory & Practice, 14,* 697–706.

Hochbaum, G. M., Sorenson, J. R., & Lorig, K. (1992). Theory in health education practice. *Health Education Quarterly, 19*(3), 295–313.

Institute of Medicine. (1988). *The Future of Public Health*. Washington, DC: National Academy Press.

Israel, B. A., Schulz, A. J., Parker, E. A., & Becker, A. B. (1998). Review of community-based research: assessing partnership approaches to improve public health. *Annual Review of Public Health, 19,* 173–202.

Kearsley, G. (1994). *Explorations in Learning & Instruction: The Theory Into Practice Database*. Available from http://tip.psychology.org/

Lancaster, B., & Roe, K. (2000). Observations of the past decade's efforts to bridge the gaps between health education and health promotion practice and research. *Health Promotion Practice, 1*(1), 33–37.

Lincoln, Y., & Guba, E. G. (1985). *Naturalistic Inquiry.* Newbury Park: Sage Publications.

Minkler, M. (2000). Using participatory action research to build healthy communities. *Public Health Reports, 115,* 191–197.

Morrissey, E., Wandersman, A., Seybolt, D., Nationa, M., Crusto, C., & Davino, K. (1997). Toward a framework for bridging the gap between science and practice in prevention: a focus on evaluator and practitioner perspectives. *Evaluation and Program Planning, 20*(3), 367–377.

Nealon, J., & Giroux, S. S. (2003). *The Theory Toolbox: Critical Concepts for the Humanities, Arts, and Social Sciences.* New York: Rowman & Littlefield Publishers, Inc.

Riley, P. L., & Kaplan, J. P. (1999). Prevention Research Centers: The Academic and Community Partnership. *American Journal of Preventive Medicine, 16*(3S), 5–6.

Schwandt, T. A. (2001). *Dictionary of Qualitative Inquiry* (2nd ed.). Thousand Oaks, CA: Sage Publications.

Sobell, L. C. (1996). Bridging the gap between scientists and practitioners: the challenge before us. *Behavior Therapy, 27,* 297–320.

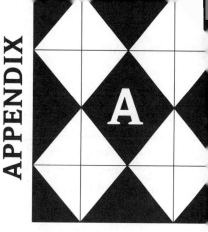

APPENDIX A

Theory or Model?

Which is it? A *theory* or a *model*? Are they different? If so, does it matter for application purposes whether we use a theory or a model or even a theoretical model? The use of these terms can, at times, become confusing, so let's try to clarify.

I discussed the meaning of the term "theory" in Chapter 1 and defined it as the end result, the outcome, the outgrowth of a dynamic process of asking and answering very specific types of questions (those concerned with causes, or "why"). I won't develop this point any further. Yet, in Chapter 1, when discussing theories and theoretical thinking, I did not talk about theoretical models. Therefore, let's now take a look at this potential synonym for "theories."

One of the best treatments of the model–theory distinction I have found consists of a chapter entitled "Theoretical Models" in the book *How to Build Social Science Theories* (Shoemaker, Tankard, & Lasorsa, 2004). In that chapter, the authors define models, carefully delineate the differences between models and theories, outline the various ways in which models can be used in social science theory building, offer a select list of criticisms scholars often make of models, and discuss different types of models. I've chosen to limit my discussion of models here to those points that are relevant for health promotion theories; if you would like a thorough, detailed treatment of the topic, I strongly recommend you look up that book.

For our purposes, it is sufficient to understand this: In its most common usage, a model consists of a representation of a given phenomenon, or reality. There are "physical models" and "conceptual models," as suggested by Shoemaker et al. (2004): "Most of us were made familiar with physical models in our childhood, when we played with miniature airplanes and miniature kitchen ovens" (p. 108).

Physical models can be made to scale (also called "scale models") or not, as in the case of models of the structure of human DNA (the famous double-helix structure).

225

In public health, we rarely work with physical models; most of the models we deal with are conceptual or mathematical. For instance, an epidemiologist attempting to map the spread of a specific virus among a population may develop a hand-drawn map with people's names in rectangles and lines with arrows connecting the various boxes, attempting to portray who caught the virus and developed the illness first, then second, third, and so forth. That same epidemiologist may work with a computer system instead, such as Geographic Information Systems (GIS; see www.gis. com) and attempt to map the epidemic across a geographical area. Moreover, epidemiologists might attempt to create mathematical models of the epidemic in an effort to predict potentially similar outbreaks in other populations. All of these are abstract representations of reality, in a "miniaturized," abstracted, even numerical form, functioning as a tool to help visualize broad phenomena.

Public health professionals who study behavior change or focus their efforts on developing prevention programs often deal with conceptual models that represent the dynamics and the relationships among certain variables at the level of the individual, community, organizations, or local and federal governments. For instance, when researchers attempt to understand which factors influence people's motivation to exercise, they may develop—based on the information gained from available scientific theories—a conceptual model similar to the one shown in Figure A–1.

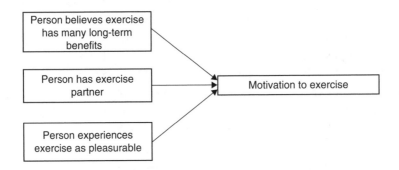

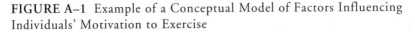

FIGURE A–1 Example of a Conceptual Model of Factors Influencing Individuals' Motivation to Exercise

It is obvious we are not representing motivation to exercise as a physical model; our model consists merely of words, boxes, and connecting arrows. These are only symbols, but with these symbols, we can represent (with limitations) the relationships among abstract constructs. Such representation can be useful in helping understand underlying mechanisms of influence and may become a useful tool when attempting to develop programs' theory of action (see Chapter 9).

If models are representations of reality, then we may conclude they are useful tools for graphically telling the story of a specific theory. That is certainly the case. We can develop a "picture" of an entire theory or select a few variables and zero-in on understanding the relationships among those few elements only. For instance, Social Cognitive Theory (SCT) has often been perceived as a complex theory, with many constructs, relationships, and theoretical propositions. Alfred McAlister, Cheryl Perry, and Guy Parcel—the authors of the chapter on Social Cognitive Theory in the Glanz book—state "SCT is very broad and ambitious, in that it seeks to provide explanations for virtually all human phenomena" (Glanz, Rimer, & Viswanath, 2008, p. 184).

Often my students complain about SCT, that it does not seem "user friendly," especially because its authors never proposed a graphic picture of the relationships among the theories' constructs. Students therefore tend to gravitate toward the Health Belief Model or the Theory of Planned Behavior because they, unlike SCT, have proposed simple diagrams of the hypothesized relationships among the variables. It's always easier to "see" abstract relationships when visual models are employed.

It would be rather simple if the term "model," therefore, was used exclusively to refer to representations (physical or conceptual, pictorial, or numeric) of phenomena or relationships. Where it becomes confusing, at times, is having the term refer to specific *theories* commonly employed in health promotion programs: the Health Belief Model; the Transtheoretical Model; the Precaution Adoption Process Model; the Ecological Model. Well, then, what are these: *models or theories?*

One way to begin distinguishing between models and theories is to bear in mind that "no matter how detailed or literal a model is, however, it is nothing more than a description of an object or process. If we want to understand how the object or process works, we need something more—a theory" (Shoemaker et al., 2004, p. 112).

Embedded in this statement we find the notion that models are somewhat "less" than theories. In its most narrow meaning, models are mere representations of a bigger reality; in its broader sense, models are theories in development. Take, for instance, the Health Belief Model (HBM). It was developed originally to address a very practical concern of its time: "to explain the widespread failure of people to participate in programs to prevent and detect disease" (tuberculosis was a specific example of one such disease) (Glanz et al., 2008, p. 46). The HBM did not develop as a set of theoretical propositions with a long history of testing before becoming the model with which we are familiar (although the model we are *now* familiar with has suffered a few modifications over time). Social psychologists employed in the U.S. Public Health Service in the 1950s developed the model in response to immediate, urgent, and practical concerns: how to motivate people to obtain important screening tests. Despite its pragmatic beginnings, the model is based on psychological theories and offers a reasonable set of theoretical propositions and explanations. Since its development, the model has been extensively tested and refined. It is, therefore, extremely difficult not to classify the HBM as a theory and to approach it merely as a model. That explains why HBM has gained "theory status" and is described in theory books, alongside SCT, but because old habits die hard, the term "model" may remain a part of its title forever. All of this to say that in health promotion practice because we tend to borrow the theories we employ from other disciplines and fields and because our concern usually centers in applying these theories (or models) to practice or research, it seems to matter little to us whether we deal with theories or with models; it seems to matter even less what labels we attach to them.

One simple way to think about the theory/model distinction is to think about theories as employees, within an organization, who enjoy substantial seniority and wisdom; models would be the new hires, the newcomers, full of fresh and innovative ideas, but lacking in experience and maturity that can only result from years of practice. Full-blown theories have survived continuous testing and refinement; models are more recent developments and propositions that still require testing and confirmation in diverse settings, but seem to work quite nicely under specific sets of contingencies.

As you attempt to contribute to the theoretical thinking efforts in public health therefore, I would recommend you begin by developing *models*. Through continuous testing and refinement, you may, after a lifetime of work, develop a robust and comprehensive theory. Start with a conceptual model (see Chapter 9 for how to use theory to ground your research questions and hypotheses). Test it yourself, and offer the model for testing by your public health colleagues. Tweak the model, based on the data obtained. Apply it to various settings and populations, then carefully craft and refine your theory.

Meanwhile, as you develop and test your own models (and potential theories), do so keeping in mind that in the field we will continue to use the terms "theory" and "model" interchangeably now and in the future without any serious consequences.

REFERENCES

Glanz, K., Rimer, B. K., & Viswanath, K. (2008). *Health Behavior and Health Education: Theory, Research, and Practice* (4th ed.). San Francisco: Jossey-Bass.

Shoemaker, P. J., Tankard Jr., J. W., & Lasorsa, D. L. (2004). *How to Build Social Science Theories*. Thousand Oaks, CA: Sage Publications.

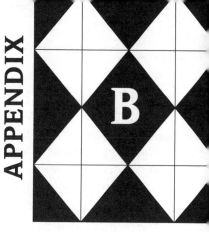

APPENDIX **B**

How to Think Theoretically

> During the last decade, there has been an acute need for theoretical innovation in the fields of population and public health. . . . In fact, there is little theory for invoking, and reflecting upon, the social and relational dimensions of public health practice. (Potvin, Gendron, Bilodeau, & Chabot, 2005, p. 591)

The quote above reflects, in essence, the underlying theme of this book: The theoretical arsenal available for use by the public health workforce is currently limited; it has been examined and found wanting. Yes, public health desperately needs more appropriate, more imaginative ways of explaining and reflecting upon its purpose and practice.

Therefore, I challenged you throughout this book to think theoretically, to begin filling in the gaps uncovered in the current theoretical landscape in health promotion. Yet I did not offer much in terms of *how to* go about developing your own theoretical thinking. In this appendix then, I wish to expose you to a few brief guidelines for thinking theoretically.

The task of developing theoretical models and further refining them into theories is complex, and I do not intend to do it justice in this short appendix; however, I do want to highlight a few available resources and provide a few "pointers" on how to get started organizing your thinking in the direction of *theory building*.

SKILLS NEEDED TO DEVELOP THEORIES

To develop your own theoretical thinking, you need a few skills in your toolbox: critical thinking skills, some knowledge or formal logic, and knowledge of your specific area of interest. When I say "critical thinking skills," I have in mind specifically the ability to assess your own thinking, to think in systematic ways, and to test the validity of your beliefs. When I refer to "formal logic," I am thinking of the capacity to identify assumptions and to "catch" when false conclusions are based on true premises. Knowledge of your specific area of interest means just that: your familiarity with the issues, existing theoretical frameworks, and the underlying mechanisms that influence, or shape, your topic of interest (be it diabetes management, smoking cessation, genetic testing, or whatever it is you are concerned about). Hopefully, these are tools you are both acquiring and sharpening throughout your professional training and your career.

GUIDELINES FOR DEVELOPING THEORY

I have in my library a couple of very useful guides for developing (and evaluating) new theories, and I believe these guides would prove helpful to you, too. One of them is a chapter in a book by Pamela Shoemaker, James William Tankard Jr., and Dominic Lasorsa (2004). The chapter titled "Using and Evaluating Theory" contains a list of 10 steps for constructing a theory. Another useful resource is the book by Dennis Mithaug (2000) titled *Learning to Theorize: A Four-Step Strategy*.

Whether you do it in 4 or 10 steps—doesn't matter how many—you can use either of these texts to guide you through the theory development (and evaluation) process. Later here, I provide a summary and my own interpretation of these guidelines; I combine recommendations from both texts and offer you my own view of the steps you need to undertake. In order therefore to begin developing your own theory, you should do the following:

1. Define the problem, issue, phenomenon, occurrence, or observation that intrigues you and has made you ask a "why" or "how" question. It does not have to be something previously uninvestigated; it might, in fact, be a phenomenon resulting from a prior research project for which you can't seem to find an already available and plausible explanation.

TIP

Dennis Mithaug (2000) suggests you begin with a discrepancy: something that should occur according to certain parameters, but doesn't. Something that doesn't "fit" the standard explanations; an anomaly, of sorts; an inconsistency between what is (what you observe) and what should be (scientists' predictions). Starting with a discrepancy can be useful because you can justify developing a new theory/model based on the inadequacies of the previous models/theories. This gives you a theoretically grounded starting point already!

2. Name the elements you identify in this problem, phenomenon, or discrepancy. Label the "parts" of your problem as best you can; these will become the constructs in your new theory/model. Remember that this step is an exercise in abstraction. Some of these "parts" may have well-known names (for instance, one element of your problem might be people's *attitudes*). Attitude has been well defined and investigated theoretically; that doesn't mean it can't be one of the elements in your new model. Because this process involves thinking abstractly, Pamela Shoemaker and her co-authors (2004) remind us that "this step can be one of the most difficult ones. Often you are trying to identify something and give it a name when no one else has identified it before" (p. 170).

TIP

When naming your constructs, think about the following:

a. Can this construct be observed?
b. Can it be measured?
c. If you're dealing with qualitative inquiry/data, can the construct vary on a scale of some sort, even if it won't be numerically measured? For example, the construct "transparency" can vary, conceptually, from "not transparent at all, or opaque" to "extremely transparent." This variation on a specific dimension (in this example, the dimension of amount, or level of transparency) will help you later establish relationships among your constructs based on their levels: "less transparency was associated, in your study, with more authoritarian leadership," for example. Establishing relationships among your constructs will be crucial for theory development.

3. Brainstorm potential causes or factors that might influence, shape, or affect your problem/phenomenon. Be creative. Don't worry about specifying the mechanisms through which the influence, shaping, or affecting takes place. Merely identify and label them (ensuring they are observable, measurable, or can be characterized on a varying dimension of some sort).

4. Begin drafting a picture or diagram of how you believe the main constructs in your theory relate to each other (Strauss, 1987, calls these pictures, "operational diagrams"). Be selective and include only the most important (and more easily measurable) constructs. Draw lines and arrows connecting related constructs. "Play" with your model/picture for a while: Try different configurations. In one model, people's self-esteem might influence their success at the workplace; in another model, try showing people's success at the workplace affecting their self-esteem. Observe your models. Talk through them, and explain them to colleagues. Do they make sense? Are they logical? Revise based on illogical or poorly defined assumptions. For instance, if your model shows people's self-esteem affecting their age, you might want to scrap that relationship from your graph (unless you're talking about psychological age, then that might be a different story). According to Strauss, this process of diagramming your theory meets several important needs, among them, "helping to pull together what you think you already know," "stimulating you to follow through with the implications of the diagram," and "clarifying what you do not know (i.e., gaps in your knowledge or understanding and so stimulating the next steps in filling [the] gaps)" (Strauss, 1987, p. 171).

5. Develop theoretical definitions for all concepts, based on a preliminary draft of your model (Shoemaker et al., 2004).

TIP

You may want to look for dictionary definitions of specific terms/ concepts, but you may also want to look to already established theories for more technical and precise definitions. You can always adapt the definition to your purposes, but available specifications can be a helpful starting point. For example, if attitude is one of the constructs in your theory, you may define it as "an opinion or way of thinking" if you use the dictionary definition of the term (The Oxford Desk Dictionary and Thesaurus—American Edition, 1997). Yet, if you research how the term is defined in social psychology, for instance, you will have available a more precise definition, one that can help you think about how you will later measure the construct (in other words, how you will operationally define attitude). According to "The Handbook of Attitudes"

> Eagly and Chaiken (1993) defined the construct as "a psychological tendency that is expressed by evaluating a particular entity with some degree of favor or disfavor (p. 1)." Accordingly, an attitude is focused on a particular entity or object, rather than all objects and situations with which it is related. Additionally, an attitude is a predisposition to like or dislike that entity, presumably with approach or avoidance consequences. (Albarracin, Johnson, & Zanna, 2005, p. 22)

6. Develop operational definitions for each construct once they have been conceptually defined (Shoemaker et al., 2004, p. 170). Remember that an operational definition consists of "complete and explicit information about how the concept will be measured" (Shoemaker et al., 2004, p. 29). In keeping with our example of the construct *attitude*, an operational definition might be "respondents' self-reports of how important they believe it is to get genetic testing, when making decisions whether to marry someone; responses will be scaled from –3 (absolutely not important) to +3 (extremely important)."

7. Begin to link the constructs in your theory with hypotheses statements. This step initiates the most complex phase of theory development—the phase in which integration of your concepts/constructs takes place, where everything starts to come together. Begin by linking constructs in pairs (two at a time; constructs A and B). Write your hypothesis for how these two constructs might relate—that is, does A affect B, or does B affect A? If A increases, does B decrease, increase, or remain unaffected? Hypothesize the nature of the relationship, the direction, the strength. Ask yourself whether other constructs (e.g., construct C) might affect the relationship between constructs A and B. If so, where does variable C come in? Does it mediate (come in between) A and B? Does it moderate the relationship (i.e., depending on what happens to C, the relationship between A and B goes in different directions)?

> **TIP**
>
> Use a matrix (a table with columns and rows) to keep track of the hypotheses you are generating (see Table B-1 for an example).

8. Provide the theoretical rationale for your proposed hypotheses (Shoemaker et al., 2004, p. 171). Explain why in each relationship each hypothesis you proposed is logical and/or evidence based.

> **TIP**
>
> If you are using a matrix such as the one in Table B-1, add the citations for all the evidence supporting your hypotheses in the matrix itself (create an additional column, specifically to list the references you are using).

9. Design a pilot study that would allow you to collect data for the variables in your theory and test your hypotheses. If you wish to conduct qualitative research or if your theory originated through qualitative inquiry, plan

Table B-1 Matrix of Hypotheses Generated When Developing a New Theory: Example

Constructs	Relationship	Direction	Mediated by	Moderated by	Hypothesis	Theoretical Rationale...
A (attitude) / B (behavior)	Correlation	—	—	C (age)	A (attitude) and B (behavior) will exhibit a statistically significant (nonzero) correlation.	The relationship between specific attitudes and behaviors is strongly supported by social psychology and health promotion theories (e.g., Theory of Planned Behavior; Social Cognitive Theory). For the proposed behavior, it has been well documented that younger adolescents espouse different attitude–behavior relationships than older adolescents (cite available research evidence here).
					The correlation between attitude and behavior will vary in strength (will be weaker or stronger), depending on the age of the persons studied (levels of C).	
D (intention to perform behavior) / B (behavior)	Causal	D → B	F (self-efficacy)	G (gender)	D (intention to perform the behavior) will determine/predict B (behavior), beyond the effects of chance (statistically significant).	The Theory of Planned Behavior proposes that intention is the strongest predictor of behavior. Nevertheless, this relationship can be modified depending on people's perceptions of the control they have over the behavior. Intentions may be strong, but if obstacles are present, the behavior may not happen as intended. Research evidence supports the notion that men and women may hold different levels of intention regarding this particular behavior (cite available research evidence here).
					The relationship will be mediated by F (self-efficacy): The strength of the association between D and B will weaken when F is considered.	
					The relationship between D and B will also vary according to gender (females will exhibit stronger intention–behavior associations than males).	

to collect data from a different sample, and use your theory's constructs to guide the analysis of these new data (as a test of the theory). Investigate whether the same theoretical relationships appear in the data from a similar sample (similar to the one used to generate the theory) and whether the relationships "hold" with samples from different population groups (e.g., if you developed your theory using, originally, a Hispanic sample, test your theory with a group of African Americans, and examine what happens to the theoretical relationships).

10. Refine your theory, based on the data from your pilot study. After you have pilot-tested your theory, carefully scrutinize the data and return to your model. Make any necessary adjustments to your hypotheses. Make note of unexpected findings, and refine your hypotheses' rationale. Remember to consider alternative explanations; sometimes we are so focused on "proving" our hypotheses we forget to investigate or consider other possibilities. After you have "tweaked" the theory to your satisfaction, design another study (or convince one of your colleagues to test your model). After *that* study, refine your theory once again, and test again and again and again.

CRITERIA FOR ASSESSING A THEORY

Once you've begun developing your theory, how will you know whether it is appropriate, relevant, and valid? How can you assess the value of this new theoretical framework? How do you know whether the story your theory tells is a good story?

Various scholars have offered criteria for judging the quality of a theory. Because this appendix is meant to be a brief exposition of this topic, I list only the most commonly used criteria here. The criteria most useful for assessing the quality of any given scientific theory (even already established and well-developed ones) are as follows:

1. Clarity and precision—the conceptual and operational definitions of the constructs are easy to understand, make sense, and connect logically; the hypothesized relationships between/among variables are unambiguous.

2. Testability—the theory can be empirically tested with relative ease. All constructs are measurable and are designed to be measured consistently across different studies.

3. Abstraction level—a theory should be applicable to many situations, groups, and circumstances. Theories that explain only a particular phenomenon, which may never reoccur, have little value. Theories should "generalize" across particular scenarios.

4. Explanatory power—this relates to the level of abstraction the theory provides and to whether it explains many different, but related, phenomena. Better theories can be applied in a wide range of contingencies (e.g., theories of motivation can explain various behaviors, from playing sports to investing money).

5. Parsimony—while theories that explain phenomena across a wide range of situations are best, the *simpler* the theory, the better it is. This criterion relates to the "clarity and precision" one mentioned previously. Simplicity and clarity tend to correlate in good theories.

6. Degree of formal development (Shoemaker et al., 2004, p. 177)—this criterion refers to how well a theory has been articulated and how much it has been tested. Formal theories have stood the test of time and faced many rounds of refinement, adjustment, and rewording; these theories are rich in details regarding the proposed relationships, measurement issues, and explanatory power. They have a dense and well-developed story to tell. Theories in developing stages lack such richness of detail, precision, and explanation.

7. Heuristic value—as Pamela Shoemaker and her colleagues (2004) remind us, "A theory is valuable when it helps us generate ideas for research and when it leads to other theoretical ideas. The more new hypotheses that can be generated from a theory, the better the theory" (p. 176).

8. Aesthetics—because theories can be beautiful, this should also be a criterion for assessing the quality of a given theory. Granted, this is a very subjective feature, yet one on which scientists have relied quite a bit (think of physicists describing their theories of the origins of the universe and how often they refer to these theories are "elegant") (Shoemaker et al., 2004).

REFERENCES

Albarracin, D., Johnson, B. T., & Zanna, M. P. (Eds.). (2005). *The Handbook of Attitudes*. Mahwah, NJ: Lawrence Erlbaum Associates.

Eagly, A. H., & Chaiken, S. (1993). *The Psychology of Attitudes*. Fort Worth, TX: Harcourt Brace Jovanovich.

Mithaug, D. E. (2000). *Learning to Theorize: A Four-Step Strategy.* Thousand Oaks: Sage Publications.

The Oxford Desk Dictionary and Thesaurus—American Edition. (1997). In F. R. Abate (Ed.). New York: Berkley Books; Oxford University Press.

Potvin, L., Gendron, S., Bilodeau, A., & Chabot, P. (2005). Integrating social theory into public health practice. *American Journal of Public health, 95,* 591–595.

Shoemaker, P. J., Tankard Jr., J. W., & Lasorsa, D. L. (2004). *How to Build Social Science Theories.* Thousand Oaks, CA: Sage Publications.

Strauss, A. L. (1987). *Qualitative Analysis for Social Scientists.* New York: Cambridge University Press.

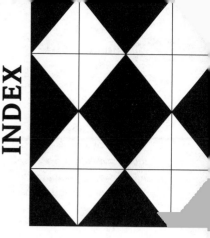

INDEX

Gottlieb, Nell H., 31, 193
Green, Lawrence W., 30
Grounded theory, 171
Guidelines, use of, 140–141

H
Habitual behavior, 115, 116
Hayden, Joanna, 78, 88, 142–143
Health Behavior and Health Education:
    Theory, Research, and Practice (Glanz,
    Rimer, & Lewis), 77, 88–89
Health Belief Model (HBM), 188–189,
    227–228
Health education
    contradiction inherent in term, 219–220
    model for, 220–221
    theoretical thinking in guidance of,
        30–34
Health promotion practice. *See* Practice
Healthy People 2010, 103, 119
Hegemony, 35–37
Historical context, of scientific theories,
    84–86, 216
Holistic treatments, 118–119
Humanistic model of health promotion,
    212, 214
Hypotheses, 83–84, 156–157, 233–235

I
Ideological takeover, prevention of, 35–37
Ideology, definition of, 35
Impact factor, 68n
Implicit theories
    application in practice, 66–68
    perception of benefits and, 38
    in program evaluation, 201–203
    in program planning, 186–187,
        194–197
Independent variables, 82–83
"individual," as term, 94
Individual responsibility for
    health, 100
Individual-level barriers, 63–64

Individual-level theories, 94–101
    alternatives to, 101–103
    bias towards, 103–105
    blind spots of, 98–100
    effectiveness of, 104
    exaggerated focus on, 90, 97–98
    incompleteness of, 100–101
    levels of theory, 93–96
Institutional level theories, 95, 96
Internal logic of programs, 186. *See also*
    Implicit theories
Interpersonal level theories, 95, 96
Intervening variables, 160
Intervention Mapping, 31, 38, 191–193
Intrapersonal level theories, 94, 95, 96,
    97–101
Introduction to Health Behavior Theory
    (Hayden), 78, 88–89, 142–143

K
Kegler, Michelle C., 77, 88
Knowledge building
    adapting processes of, 216–218
    scientific model of, 217
Kok, Gerjo, 31, 193
Kreuter, Marshall W., 30

L
Language, in shaping reality, 6
Latent variable, 81
Lewis, Frances Marcus, 77
Linear theories
    alternative to, 132–136
    data analyses and, 130–132
    description of, 124–125
    dynamic approaches compared to,
        128–129
    exaggerated focus on, 90, 124–125
Locus of control, 84

M
Mathematical models, 226
Meaning